MW01132847

WOMEN AND GUT HEALTH

STOP LIVING IN SILENCE, SUFFERING, AND STIGMAS
WITH YOUR GASTROINTESTINAL ISSUES AND PLAN
FOR IMPROVED, SYMPTOM-FREE DIGESTION AND
OVERALL WELL-BEING

J. JOHNSON

CONTENTS

INTRODUCTION

How's your poop? It's not exactly a topic of conversation to have with friends or family; it's too personal and unpleasant. Women don't want to talk about their gut-related problems due to the associated stigma. Talking about gut problems like diarrhea, gas, bloating, constipation, or abdominal pain can be embarrassing and shameful.

There's fear of having an accident on yourself from frequent bouts of diarrhea. You worry when that smell from uncontrolled passing gas is offensive. Bloating, constipation, and abdominal pain can stop you in your tracks if severe enough and can consequently interrupt work or going about daily life.

Do you know if your poop is normal or not? Or do you just wipe yourself, flush the toilet, and get out of the bathroom as quickly as possible without really looking at your stool in the toilet? I have to admit I can be uncomfortable embracing this conversation as well. I don't like to have bowel movements in public bathrooms unless I really have to or I am the only one there. I prefer to wait until I am in the privacy of my own bathroom. In the past, I never talked to anybody about any gut problems and vice versa. However, I learned my lesson the hard way. Women shouldn't ignore gut problems, thinking it's just a part of being "normal," "female," or "just waiting for the problem to pass."

Persistent gut problems can lead to more serious digestive conditions such as irritable bowel syndrome (IBS) or ulcerative colitis. Gut health is too important to be ignored, especially if you are seeking to

- alleviate the gut problems disrupting your life.
- improve your overall health and well-being, i.e., better sleep, increased energy, balanced mood, and freedom from pain.

In the beginning, these problems may seem overwhelming with no solution in sight. When it comes to improving your gut health, where do you begin? How do you know if you have good gut health in the first place? If you don't have it, how do you get it and maintain it?

Have you ever experienced bloating, constipation, stomach cramps, or other digestive issues? If so, you are not alone. In fact, more than 20 million Americans suffer from some form of chronic digestive disorder each year (GI Alliance, 2021). It can be incredibly uncomfortable and even embarrassing to talk about these issues, which is why learning about the subject can be so beneficial. Understanding more about digestive health can give us the tools we need to take better care of ourselves.

Are you familiar with women's digestive health? If so, then you may already know that it is a subject of vital importance. However, if you are not sure what it is all about or why it matters, then this book can help explain exactly why.

It's easy to overlook the importance of women's digestive health. Yet, it is vitally important for our well-being and overall quality of life. This book covers everything from the basics of digestion to how to improve specific disorders. There is information about nutrient absorption and how different types of food affect our digestion.

We also learn about signs that might indicate an underlying issue that requires medical attention. You'll gain insight into the latest research involving women's digestive health and even get tips on lifestyle changes that can improve your overall well-being.

There's no need to feel overwhelmed by the topic. This book provides a friendly entry point for anyone looking for more information on a woman's digestive health. With its easy-to-understand explanations and detailed facts backed by current research, this book takes an approachable approach to a common but often overlooked topic in women's healthcare.

Not only will you learn more about the basics of how your digestive system works, but you'll also get a deep dive into some of the common conditions that can affect this important body system. From learning about IBS and other digestive issues to discovering natural remedies for improving digestion, this book has something for everyone!

This book provides an accessible way to learn more about how dietary choices and lifestyle habits can play a big role in keeping your digestive system healthy. And now that we know just how essential women's digestive health is to our overall wellness, there's never been a better time to take a deeper look into what's going on inside our bodies.

After reading this book, takeaways for women are:

- learn the concept of gut health and its vital importance
- understand poop despite stigmatized matters
- anatomical and physiological reasons why women have more gut problems than men
- gut-related symptoms unique to women and other symptoms not to be ignored
- how to self-advocate to get the best care
- what kind of innovations in gut health research can be expected in years to come

It's time for women to be silent no more and speak up for the best care they deserve. Your gut will take care of you if you pay attention and take care of it.

As a nurse with over 40 years of experience in the healthcare industry, I am uniquely qualified to provide advice on women's digestive health. I have spent many years working in a day surgery unit where I provided caring and compassionate support to my patients who came in weekly for gastrointestinal (GI) procedures. During my time in this role, I gained valuable insights into digestive health issues that are common among women.

This wealth of experience has enabled me to become an authority on the subject. I am passionate about helping women achieve and maintain good gut health without feeling any stigma or shame about it. As someone who has seen first-hand how digestive health issues can affect a person's quality of life, I strive to impart knowledge that will help others understand how they can take control of their own health.

My comprehensive understanding of the science behind digestion allows me to explain complex topics in a way that is simple yet detailed. Additionally, I also use real-world examples whenever possible so that readers can better relate to the information I provide. Above all else, it is my goal to inspire people by providing them with the tools and resources they need in order to make positive changes when it comes to their own digestive health.

Over the years, I have come to value evidence-based approaches over popular trends. Research-backed nutrition can truly benefit our bodies when done properly. My goal is to provide you with the tools and facts you need to make healthy decisions about your specific digestive concerns without having to blindly follow every trend out there.

Overall, I'm writing this because I want to share my knowledge and experience so that other women can benefit from the information I have to offer. I have an extensive education in nutrition and biology, so I understand how food affects our bodies, as well as how to create balanced approaches to healthy eating. In the end, though, my passion for women's digestive health came from my own personal struggles with it in my own life, which has led me to help other women who suffer from digestive issues as well.

As with any medical advice or opinion that I provide in this book, it's always important that you discuss anything you're considering trying with your doctor first. Talking to a trusted physician about your experiences, concerns, and habits will help you determine what's best for you and how you can best tackle it.

At the same time, I'm providing detailed scientific explanations about digestion in this book, along with evidence-based tips backed by reliable research. I also strive to provide practical ways readers can implement dietary changes that might improve their digestive health in a way they can really understand. To do this effectively requires going beyond just giving facts but rather explaining why those facts are important so that readers get a better overall understanding of how digestion works.

I have been through this experience as well. I understand what it feels like to be concerned about one's own digestive health. This book is my way of helping other women gain the confidence and understanding they need to take control of their own well-being. With this guide in hand, I am confident that any woman can learn more about her digestive system and make informed decisions for a healthier gut. So, if you're ready to take charge of your digestive health and make positive changes, start reading this book today! You won't regret it.

1

WHAT'S GUT HAVE TO DO WITH IT? EVERYTHING!

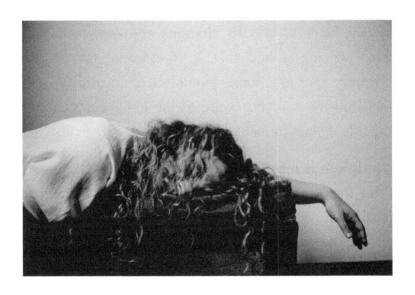

I f you ask or research "gut health" you will find different interpretations of what it means. The most important fact about gut health is that it's vital to your overall health and well-being.

You likely already know some information and facts about gut health. For instance, you're probably aware that the food you eat can affect your poop and pooping habits. You may also know that the gut microbiome is an integral part of digestive health. Gut health has been a hot topic in recent years, and for good reason.

However, did you know that the digestive system is crucial to our immune system and helps us fight off pathogens? Did you also know that our digestive system helps us absorb vitamins and minerals from what we ingest and that it is essential for proper hormone production, blood detoxification, and metabolism? Are you aware of the brain-gut axis and the role it plays in mental well-being?

Gut health is more than just a trendy topic; it's something that everyone should pay attention to—women in particular. Women have unique challenges that can affect their gut health, including pregnancy and hormonal changes related to menstruation or menopause—crucial factors that also affect our gut health.

It's important to understand that the food you consume impacts your gut microbiome. This microbiome has a direct effect on your health, both physically and mentally. Foods that are packed with unhealthy fats, processed sugars, and preservatives can disrupt the balance of your gut microbiome, leading to a host of health issues. In this chapter, we'll discuss the different aspects of gut health and why women should be particularly attentive to their own gut health. Let's start by looking at the different components that make up a healthy gut.

WHAT IS GUT HEALTH?

Gut health is defined by the World Health Organization (WHO) as the well-being of an individual's digestive system (Bischoff, 2011). It includes a wide range of elements, such as the balance of microorganisms in the gut, which is essential for effective digestion and absorption. The microbial diversity in our gut affects almost every aspect of our health, from our metabolism and immune system to our mood and cognition. When it comes to promoting good gut health, a beneficial, well-rounded diet plays a key role.

Why Is Gut Health Important?

Gut health is incredibly important for women, as it impacts many aspects of overall health and well-being.

Good gut health is associated with a stronger immune system, reduced inflammation, and better digestion, as well as improved mood and deeper sleep. A healthy gut also plays a role in hormone balance, reproductive health, and skin health.

The gut houses trillions of bacteria, fungi, and other microorganisms collectively known as the microbiome. These microbes help break down food and extract nutrients while playing a role in healthy gut barrier function. Poor gut health has been linked to a range of issues like food sensitivities, autoimmune diseases, and digestive disorders such as IBS (Dix, 2018).

Women's bodies are especially sensitive to changes in their microbiome because of hormonal fluctuations that occur during the menstrual cycle. Hormonal imbalances can disrupt the delicate microbiome balance, leading to issues like bloating or fatigue after eating certain foods. For example, high levels of progesterone can cause an overgrowth of bad bacteria in the gut, leading to digestive issues (Hi & Li, 2021).

Also, low levels of estrogen can weaken the mucus barrier in the gut, making it more difficult for beneficial bacteria to do their job (Paone & Cani, 2020). Therefore, it's so important for women to prioritize a balanced diet rich in probiotic-rich fermented foods like yogurt or kefir that feed the beneficial bacteria in their guts and promote healthy microbial diversity.

In addition to dietary changes, regular exercise can also support good intestinal function by promoting blood flow to the digestive tract and helping move food through the body more quickly. Stress reduction techniques can also help keep hormones balanced, which supports better absorption of key micronutrients needed for optimal gut health. Together with these lifestyle modifications, probiotic supplements may help restore the delicate balance of microorganisms, especially when taken regularly over time.

What Don't We Know About Gut Health?

From a scientific perspective, gut health is complex. Despite the significant advances in our understanding of gut health, there are still many unanswered questions. For example, we still do not know why some individuals suffer from GI disorders while others remain unaffected. We also lack information regarding the long-term effects of certain treatments and dietary interventions on gut health.

Additionally, we need more in-depth, specific information to determine the exact gender-specific differences in the composition or functioning of the human microbiome and how these factors might influence overall health. For women specifically, there is a need for more research into how hormones may affect gut health and how the microbiome may be shaped by menstrual cycles, pregnancy, and menopause.

It remains unclear if diet can modify the microbiome and reduce symptoms associated with medical conditions experienced by women, such as endometriosis or polycystic ovarian syndrome. Finally, little is known about how environmental factors such as stress can impact a woman's microbiome and her risk of developing certain diseases or conditions.

In sum, we have a lot of information available. However, tying it together and understanding each part's specific influence on women's health remains a challenge. What is known, however, is that the gut microbiome has a profound influence on overall health and well-being, and being more aware of our changes can help add to the wealth of knowledge out there.

THE PLAIN BASICS OF DIGESTION

It all starts with digestion. It is generally accepted that it takes anywhere from 24 to 72 hours for food to pass through the digestive system, depending on the individual and the type of food being eaten. During this process, food is broken down into smaller pieces, and nutrients are extracted from it. The intestines, stomach, pancreas, gallbladder, and other organs work together in a complex series of steps to digest our food.

Digestion begins in the mouth as we chew and break down food particles into smaller chunks. Smaller chunks can be easily absorbed by the body and will move further along the digestive tract. Then the food moves through the esophagus and enters the stomach, where powerful acids and enzymes break them down even further.

The food is pushed into the small intestine, where important macronutrients like proteins, vitamins, carbohydrates, fats, and minerals are absorbed. The now partially digested material gets pushed into the large intestine or colon, where water and electrolytes are removed from it. Then it will enter your rectum, where it becomes stool or poop.

In summary, digestion occurs when food passes from our mouths all the way through our system until waste products are eliminated at last. This complex digestion process involves different organs such as our teeth for chewing, throat for swallowing, esophagus for transporting food, and stomach for breaking down nutrients. It also involves the pancreas for producing digestive juices, liver for producing bile, and small intestine for absorption. Also, we have the large intestine for storage of waste products and the rectum for defecation, etc., all playing their important part in aiding the absorption of essential macronutrients.

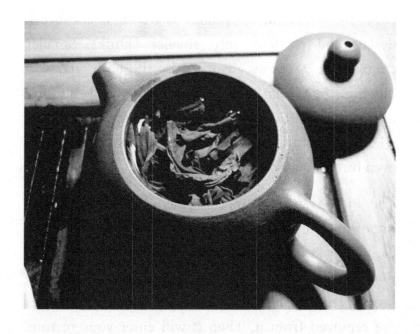

What Is Responsible for Your Gut Working Properly?

The gut is an incredibly complex ecosystem that requires many elements to work properly. First and foremost, it relies on the microbiome. The microbiome is a mix of trillions of bacteria, viruses, and fungi that live in your digestive system. It's estimated that your body has up to 10 times more microbes than human cells. These microbes play an important role in keeping your gut working properly. They help us break down food, absorb nutrients, protect us from bad bacteria and viruses, and a host of other functions.

Additionally, healthy digestion depends on the release of hormones like gastrin, secretin, and cholecystokinin. These hormones help coordinate the activities of the digestive system. The muscles in our intestines also play an important role by contracting rhythmically to move food through the digestive tract. Finally, our brains can affect how well our guts function—when we're stressed out or anxious, our guts are less effective at digesting food. In short, it takes all these components working together for your gut to work properly.

How Does the Microbiome Work?

The microbiome comprises both good and bad bacteria —the majority being beneficial bacteria. The microbiome is a complex and diverse community of microorganisms that live on and inside the human body. It is estimated that our bodies are home to over 100 trillion microbes, including bacteria, viruses, protozoa, and fungi. The bulk of these microbes are found in the gut, where they form a unique ecosystem known as the gut microbiome.

The gut microbiome plays an important role in helping us digest food, breaking down complex molecules into ones that can be easily absorbed by the body. Good bacteria help digest food, produce certain vitamins, regulate metabolism and detoxification processes, and play an essential role in immune system development. The bad bacteria can lead to inflammation, infections, and diseases such as Crohn's disease, inflammatory bowel disease (IBD), or IBS.

Furthermore, it helps regulate the immune system by preventing harmful bacteria from taking hold in the intestines. It also produces short-chain fatty acids, which act as a source of energy for cells lining the digestive tract. Additionally, it synthesizes vitamins and other essential nutrients that help keep our bodies functioning optimally.

The microbiome is constantly changing due to factors like diet, lifestyle choices, medications, and age. Interactions between different species of bacteria allow for beneficial traits to be passed on from one generation to another and ensure that the microbiome remains healthy and balanced. To ensure optimal health, it's important to maintain a balanced diet rich in fiber and probiotics—these are living organisms found in fermented foods such as yogurt or kimchi, which have been linked to improved digestion and absorption of nutrients in humans.

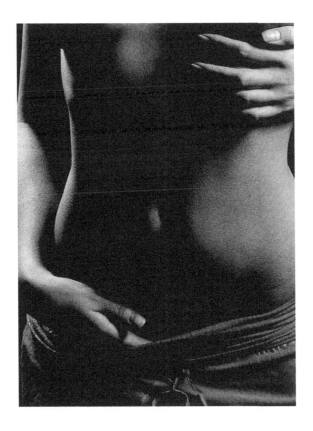

Overall, the microbiome plays an incredibly important role in maintaining our overall health by helping us digest food properly and absorb all its necessary nutrients, fighting off disease-causing pathogens, regulating immune responses, or aiding metabolism processes. It can also play a role in controlling weight gain and

obesity, preventing allergies, protecting against inflammation, improving cognitive function, influencing
moods, and even helping with skin conditions like acne.

In conclusion, while we're still learning about how the
microbiome functions within our bodies, it's clear that
having a healthy balance of bacteria is crucial for
overall well-being. By eating right and supplementing
with probiotics when necessary, we can keep our
microbiomes happy.

WHAT CONTRIBUTING FACTORS AFFECT THE GUT?

There are several factors that can affect the gut and its
microbiome. There is no one problem that affects the
gut. Rather, it is a combination of factors, including
diet, lifestyle, medications, and age.

Diet is a big factor in gut problems and symptoms.
Eating processed and sugary foods, as well as unhealthy
fats, can lead to inflammation in the gut. This inflammation can cause digestive distress, bloating, gas, and
abdominal cramps. Eating too much or too little can
also cause digestive issues. Drinking plenty of water is
essential for good digestion. Dehydration can lead to
constipation and other GI problems.

Sleep also plays a role in digestive health. Not getting enough sleep disrupts hormones and the body's ability to process food properly. Stress can also trigger digestive issues by interfering with hormone regulation and inflammation levels. Chronic stress has been linked to conditions like IBS, heartburn, and ulcers.

Inflammation is another common factor behind many gut issues. Chronic inflammation interferes with normal digestion processes and can cause pain and discomfort in the stomach (Pahwa & Jialal, 2019). Hormonal imbalances are also linked to digestion problems (Women and Gut Health, n.d.). Changes in hormones due to pregnancy, menopause, or specific medications can affect how your body processes food. Finally, age can affect the microbiome and digestive health in several ways. As we get older, our bodies struggle to process food, and our microbiome is more likely to be imbalanced.

Certain medications can also disrupt the microbiome and affect digestion. Antibiotics, for example, kill both beneficial and harmful bacteria in the gut, resulting in digestive distress, bloating, and constipation. Additionally, medications for conditions like depression or anxiety can affect the microbiome and lead to digestive issues.

As you can see, many factors of life can affect and disrupt the gut and its microbiome. However, in most cases, intentional lifestyle choices and changes to diet can help restore balance and help maintain optimal digestive health.

By understanding the factors that contribute to gut problems and symptoms, you can make lifestyle changes that support your digestive system.

Signs of a Healthy Gut

When your gut is in balance, you should feel comfortable after eating and have regular bowel movements. Your energy level should be consistent throughout the day, and you should have no digestive issues or pain. Additionally, a healthy microbiome can help improve immunity, aid in digestion, reduce inflammation, and keep hormones balanced. Other signs of a healthy gut include

- clear skin
- mental clarity and focus
- consistent energy levels throughout the day
- healthy weight and appetite regulation
- strong immunity
- regular elimination without pain or bloating

While these signs might seem minuscule, they show how vital a healthy gut is to our overall well-being, as it can influence our physical and mental health. Given the importance of a healthy gut, you should strive to maintain your digestive health every day. Doing so will lead you to a healthier life and enjoy all the benefits that come with it.

THE GUT AND ITS RELATION TO PHYSICAL AND MENTAL WELL-BEING

A healthy gut is essential for maintaining overall physical and mental well-being. Our digestive system is home to trillions of microorganisms that play a vital role in helping us digest our food and ward off disease-causing pathogens. Having a healthy gut can improve our energy levels, mood, brain health, and more.

A strong hormone system is one of the most important benefits of having a healthy gut. Our hormones regulate our bodily functions, including digestion and metabolism (Women and Gut Health, n.d.). When our gut isn't working properly, it can lead to an imbalance in these hormones, which can cause various problems such as weight gain or digestion issues. By maintaining a balanced gut microbiome, we can ensure that our hormonal levels remain balanced and help us stay healthy.

Heart health is another benefit of having a healthy gut. Studies have shown that people with higher levels of healthy bacteria in their guts are less likely to suffer from heart disease than those who don't have the same amount of bacteria in their guts (Cryan et al., 2019). A balanced gut flora helps reduce inflammation and cholesterol levels in the blood, which helps keep the heart healthy.

Brain health is also intimately linked to the state of our gut health. The connection between the two has been referred to as the "gut-brain axis." Some research evidence suggests that an unhealthy microbiome can contribute to anxiety, depression, bipolar disorder, and other mental health conditions (Cryan et al., 2019). A healthy balance of beneficial bacteria can help promote feelings of calmness and relaxation by sending signals to our brains via our vagus nerve, which connects the digestive tract with the brainstem.

Improved moods are another significant benefit that comes with having a balanced microbiome in our gut. Certain strains of beneficial bacteria produce serotonin —often referred to as "the happy hormone"—which helps fight symptoms associated with depression or anxiety, such as insomnia or irritability. Additionally, they also reduce inflammation throughout the body, which can also lift your spirits.

Healthy sleep is another outcome of having a balanced microbiome. Not only does it promote better sleep quality, but research has also shown that it reduces fatigue during waking hours too. Additionally, if you struggle with stress or worry, then having an abundance of beneficial bacteria will help calm your mind so you get into deep restorative sleep at nighttime without any difficulty!

Balanced digestion is yet another important aspect when it comes to having a healthy gut. Good quality probiotics help reduce symptoms associated with IBS, such as bloating or abdominal pain, while also providing greater nutrient absorption from foods eaten throughout the day.

Having a balanced weight can also come along with maintaining good gut health. Certain strains within your microbes will actually help break down fats present within foods so they're easier for you to digest. This not only reduces any unwanted weight gain, but it also keeping you fuller for longer periods, so you don't overindulge on snacks throughout the day.

Increased energy levels are yet another great example, as improved digestion means nutrients are more easily absorbed, meaning more energy is available for cell growth or production and general maintenance processes around this area. This eliminates feelings of sluggishness and lethargy throughout each day.

Clear skin is one ultimate benefit. Some studies have found that those who maintain good balances within their microbiomes tend to have healthier-looking skin than those whose flora isn't quite up to par (Cryan et al., 2019). This could be due to reduced inflammation caused by imbalances or improved nutrient uptake meaning cells regenerate quicker and healthier than usual—much like how better hydration also leads to clear complexions.

Finally, decreased inflammation throughout the body occurs when your microbiome remains balanced. This could be due to improved uptake or breakdown rates on certain nutrients (including fats) or increased production and activation rates on some anti-inflammatory chemicals held within certain bacterial species' genomes. Either way, it's important for overall wellbeing and should not be overlooked when considering all things related to improving one's own health.

GUT HEALTH IN THE UNITED STATES TODAY

The rise of gut symptoms and conditions in the United States population has been a stark reminder of how big of an impact our digestive health can have on our overall well-being. Gut issues are becoming increasingly more common, with millions of Americans being affected each year. People can experience a variety of different symptoms, such as abdominal pain, bloating, nausea, constipation, diarrhea, and fatigue (Bäckhed et al., 2012). Additionally, some people may develop more severe conditions such as celiac disease or IBD.

The rise of these concerns is a worrying reality that many people are facing. While there can be many causes and contributing factors, they all have one thing in common—women are more prone to them than men. In fact, over 100 million women in the United States are living with gut issues, often treating them as a "normal" part of life (Reddy, 2022).

It's unclear exactly why digestive diseases continue to rise, but some experts think it has something to do with changes in our diets and lifestyles. In fact, there isn't just one factor that causes these kinds of issues, but rather a multitude of environmental, dietary, and lifestyle-related factors that all contribute in different ways. Consequently, it can often be difficult to pinpoint the true cause.

Over the past few decades, we've seen an increase in processed foods and sugary snacks, which can contribute to digestion problems like IBS. Most people have diets packed with processed foods full of unhealthy chemicals like pesticides and genetically modified organisms (GMOs). Such a diet is known as the Standard American Diet (SAD), and it leads to an imbalance of gut bacteria, which causes dysbiosis and decreased immunity. It's also no secret that Americans are often under high levels of stress, exposing them to greater risks for GI issues (Dix, 2018).

Additionally, stress levels have gone up due to jobs becoming more demanding and technology making it hard for us to unplug from work or school. All these factors combined can lead to worse gut health. Besides diet and lifestyle changes, genetics may also play a role. People might inherit certain genes that make them more susceptible to digestive problems like Crohn's disease or ulcerative colitis.

That's why it's important to improve your overall health if you're suffering from any kind of digestive issue or discomfort. By doing so, you can help reduce your risk for further problems down the line. Eating whole foods in combination with regular exercise and adequate sleep are essential components of a healthy lifestyle. These habits will provide your body with the essential nutrients it needs while helping you maintain a balanced gut microbiome.

In addition, limiting exposure to toxins and pollutants can also help prevent many common GI problems from ever arising in the first place. Even if you're already experiencing discomfort or symptoms related to poor gut health, making simple changes such as these can still improve things significantly over time while reducing your risk for further complications down the road.

It's clear that poor gut health not only affects how we feel physically but mentally as well—people with gut problems often suffer from depression and anxiety due to their inability to eat certain foods or their changing dietary needs over time.

We need to be aware of our own digestive health and take steps toward optimizing it by eating healthy foods and maintaining good hydration levels while also managing stress levels through activities like yoga or meditation. By following these steps, we can reduce the chances of developing more serious digestive issues down the line while also creating a happier life overall.

Top 10 Digestion and Gut Health Myths and the Truth

Digestive and gut health can be a topic of concern for many women. There are numerous myths and misconceptions about the digestive system and gut health that make it difficult to figure out what is true and what is not. In this section, we will explore the top 10 myths and the truth about digestion and gut health to help women better understand their digestive systems.

Myth 1: You need to have a bowel movement every day.

- Truth: The frequency of bowel movements can vary from person to person, and every woman's body is different. While some women may have a bowel movement every day, others may only have one every two or three days. It's important to pay attention to your body and try to establish a regular pattern that works for you.

Myth 2: You can "cleanse" your gut with a detox diet.

- Truth: There's no evidence to support the idea that a detox diet or cleanse will improve gut health. In fact, some of these diets can be harmful and disrupt the natural balance of bacteria in your gut. It's best to have a healthy, well-rounded diet to promote your best gut health.

Myth 3: Peppermint oil cures digestive issues.

- Truth: While peppermint oil may ease symptoms like bloating and gas, it's not a cure for digestive issues. It's important to consult

with a healthcare provider to determine the
underlying cause of digestive issues and
develop a treatment plan.

Myth 4: Gluten-free diets are healthier.

- Truth: Gluten-free diets are only necessary for
  people who have celiac disease or gluten
  sensitivity, but for others, there's no evidence
  that a gluten-free diet is healthier. A good deal
  of gluten-free products are actually less healthy
  than their gluten-containing counterparts and
  may be higher in calories, sugar, and fat.

Myth 5: Probiotics are always beneficial.

- Truth: While some probiotics may be beneficial
  for gut health, not all probiotics are created
  equal. Different strains of bacteria have
  different effects on the gut, and not all
  probiotics have been studied extensively. It's
  important to talk to a healthcare provider
  before taking probiotics.

Myth 6: Dairy products cause digestive issues.

- Truth: While some people may be lactose intolerant and can't tolerate dairy products, others can digest them without any issues. Dairy products are a good source of calcium and other important nutrients, so it's important to talk to a healthcare provider before eliminating them from your diet.

Myth 7: Fiber supplements are just as good as fiber from food.

- Truth: While fiber supplements can help increase fiber intake, they don't provide the same benefits as fiber from food. Whole foods contain a variety of nutrients that are important for gut health, so it's important to get fiber from a variety of sources.

Myth 8: It's normal to experience bloating after meals.

- Truth: Occasional bloating after meals is normal, but frequent or severe bloating may be a sign of an underlying digestive issue. It's important to talk to a healthcare provider if you experience frequent or severe bloating.

Myth 9: Drinking water with meals interferes with digestion.

- Truth: Drinking water with meals can actually aid in digestion by helping to break down food. It can also help move it through the digestive system. It's important to stay hydrated throughout the day, including during meals.

Myth 10: Stress doesn't affect gut health.

- Truth: Stress can have a significant impact on gut health. Stress can disrupt the balance of bacteria in the gut and lead to digestive issues. It's important to manage stress through strategies like exercise, meditation, and therapy to maintain good gut health.

Myth 11: Your stomach shrinks if you eat less.

- Truth: Although it may feel like your stomach shrinks when you eat less, that's not the case. Instead, smaller meals can train your body to feel full sooner and reduce hunger. Eating balanced meals throughout the day can help with weight management and maintain a healthy digestive system.

Myth 12: It takes seven years to digest gum.

- Truth: Chewing gum does not actually get digested, so it doesn't stay in your digestive system for seven years. Instead, the gum passes through the body and is eliminated in feces. However, it's still important to practice moderation when chewing gum, as it can cause digestive issues if consumed in large amounts.

Overall, there are many myths and misconceptions about digestion and gut health that can make it difficult to know what's true and what's not. By understanding the truth about these top 10 myths, women can take control of their digestive health and feel their best. Remember to talk to a healthcare provider if you have any concerns about your gut health.

MY SURVEY

I conducted a random survey using information from the day surgery area of a hospital logbook of patients coming in for GI procedures over four weeks. Out of the total 80 patients studied during this period, 59 were female and 21 were male, making it almost a 2:1 ratio. The common complaints reported by these patients included abdominal pain, dysphagia, heartburn, and rectal bleeding.

GI symptoms may sometimes indicate an underlying medical condition that warrants further examination and treatment. Some symptoms noticed could include bloating, constipation, diarrhea, heartburn, nausea, and vomiting. If these issues persist or worsen over time, then it is advised to consult with a medical professional instead of ignoring them.

Our survey focused on GI-related issues along with gender division among such cases to get a better understanding of the same. From our findings, we can clearly see that females have been more prone to such diseases than males, yet both genders need to take precautionary measures as soon as they experience them to avoid any future complications or health risks. The nurses and doctors in our day surgery area are always there to help if one needs any advice regarding gut-related issues or anything else specific to their condition.

SUCCESS STORY

According to Linda (2022) from Just for Tummies, Deborah, a busy working woman, had been battling digestive health issues for years. However, the loss of her dear mother put her under immense emotional stress, and her symptoms spiked alarmingly. The once sporadic symptoms of nausea, diarrhea, stomach gurgling, upper abdominal pain, and acid reflux turned constant and intolerable, causing her immense distress and discomfort (Linda, 2022b).

Suffering from constant diarrhea led to extensive weight loss despite Deborah's already slim stature. Adding to her woes, some food items suddenly started triggering severe reactions, and her diet became significantly restricted. Determined to find answers and relief, Deborah sought the help of various digestive health experts, pouring thousands of dollars into countless consultations and overwhelming supplement recommendations. Despite her efforts, none of these solutions seemed to make even a minor difference to her critical condition.

In her desperate yet persevering search for a solution, Deborah stumbled upon Just for Tummies, a company dedicated to gut health, helmed by Linda Booth, a renowned digestive health expert. Intrigued by the promising success stories of other patients, Deborah got in touch with Linda, hoping her expertise and tailored supplements could finally provide her much-awaited respite.

Linda, after closely assessing Deborah's condition, recommended a five-day cleanse to tackle the persistent diarrhea. Skeptical after her numerous failed attempts with other treatments, Deborah hesitantly embraced the cleanse under Linda's guidance. Much to her disbelief and delight, the cleanse did wonders for Deborah. Her incessant diarrhea problem steadily alleviated as the days passed, and she began to regain control over her daily life. The newfound relief lifted her spirits and restored her faith in the possibility of regaining her health and vitality by finally addressing the root causes of her digestive issues and curating a plan tailored to her needs.

From there, she could relieve her stress, heal her gut, and repair her digestion. She could rebuild the strength of her immune system, improve her nutrition absorption, and reduce overall inflammation. Deborah's story is a testament to the power of healing the gut with natural remedies and personalized care—it can transform lives.

Our gut health is often overlooked and underestimated. Deborah's story inspires others struggling with digestive issues to never give up in their pursuit of relief and well-being. With determination, perseverance, and the aid of the right specialist, anyone can reclaim control over their health and, in turn, their life.

REFLECTION QUESTIONS

- What are some common gut issues that you face?
- How do you think a healthy diet can improve your overall gut health?
- What preventative measures are most effective for keeping your gut in good shape?
- What tips do you have for people who are trying to better manage their gut health?
- What lifestyle changes can you make now to help improve your digestive system?
- What warning signs should you look out for that could indicate a possible gut health issue?

2

WE DON'T WANT TO TALK ABOUT
IT BUT WE MUST: POOP

Pooping is a perfectly natural process, yet it carries with it a certain stigma due to its often-unpleasant odor and the fact that it is associated with bodily waste. The term "stigma" comes from the Latin word for mark or brand, and it generally refers to an attribute of something that separates it from other things negatively. With pooping, there are a variety of reasons our society views this activity as distasteful.

For starters, poop is simply unpleasant. It smells bad and can look unappealing in certain situations, which leads people to associate this natural function with being dirty and gross. Some cultural norms may dictate that talking about pooping should be avoided in polite company. So, even if we know that everyone poops, we still feel uncomfortable discussing the subject openly.

The awkwardness around this natural bodily process fuels the stigmas.

The shame associated with pooping even extends to language: many people refer to poop by less-than-savory terms like "crap" or "boo-boo" rather than its more clinical name (feces). In some way, these childish names can be less embarrassing than their technical counterparts.

Finally, there is also a bit of hypocrisy involved when it comes to pooping. While most people agree poop is gross, they will still have no problem talking about their own bowel movements in detail or indulging in bathroom humor at inappropriate times! This paradox allows us all to laugh at our own bodily functions while simultaneously shaming others for engaging in them—an attitude that further reinforces the stigma surrounding pooping.

All of this means that despite being something we all do every day without thinking twice about it, pooping is still seen as something that should never be talked about or discussed openly. Yet despite its shameful reputation, pooping remains an essential bodily function; understanding its importance and demystifying some of its misconceptions can help reduce the stigma surrounding this commonly performed activity!

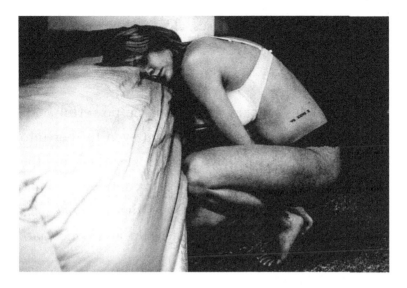

PHYSIOLOGY OF POOPING

Poop. Crap. Boo-boo. #2. BM. Defecation. Shit—when it comes to talking about the subject, it's no wonder why there is so much stigma attached to this bodily function. But, in reality, there is no need for all the shame and embarrassment because pooping is just a natural part of everyday life—an experience that every single human being does.

So what exactly goes into making poop? The digestion process starts in the mouth when you begin to chew your food. Your saliva contains enzymes that help break down carbohydrates into simpler forms like glucose. As you continue to chew, the food is mashed up and mixed with more saliva before it's swallowed in small chunks called boluses. The bolus then travels through your esophagus—a long tube between your throat and stomach—to your stomach (Tresca, 2003).

Once the bolus reaches your stomach, powerful acids and enzymes start to break it down even further into smaller particles so they can be absorbed by the intestines later on. The stomach also contracts periodically to mix and churn up these digested particles before pushing the mixture out again as chyme (partially digested food; Tresca, 2003).

After passing from the stomach, chyme enters the small intestine, where most nutrient absorption happens through its walls. Here, two main pancreas-produced juices are secreted: pancreatic juice, rich in enzymes that break down proteins, fats, and starch; and bile, produced in the liver, which emulsifies fat droplets so they're easier to digest. Throughout this process of breaking down nutrients further, digestive juices mix with chyme, causing it to become more watery until what's left is called intestinal juice, which is eventually passed out through defecation (Tresca, 2003).

Finally, after passing through both small and large intestines, what's left of undigested material makes its way to the rectum where it gets stored until defecated through peristalsis (involuntary wavelike muscle contractions; Tresca, 2003).

It's truly amazing how our bodies take what we eat and break it down into fuel for our bodies. But don't forget that not all of what we eat ends up as poop—some of it actually gets recycled back into our system. So while you may see a lot of waste coming out when you go to the bathroom, rest assured that your body puts a lot of effort into breaking down that food so that you can get those necessary nutrients.

TYPES OF POOP

Pooping is a regular and necessary part of life. It's the body's way of eliminating waste from the system, but it can also tell us a lot about our health. When we don't poop regularly or when something looks "off" about it, it could be a sign that something else is going on in the body.

Looking at your poop can provide important clues to your health and well-being, such as providing evidence of dehydration, nutrient deficiencies, inflammation, infections, food sensitivities, and more. While pooping may not be a favorite topic of conversation, under-standing what goes into making good number twos is important for optimal gut health.

So let's talk poop! Color and texture are two key factors in determining if you have healthy poops. What should you be looking out for? Healthy poops are usually brown or light brown in color with an earthy smell (yes, there should always be an aroma to your business) because they contain bacteria and small amounts of substances like bilirubin that give them their color.

A healthy poop will also have a thick consistency like toothpaste—if it's too liquidy, then that could indicate diarrhea or another issue. On the other hand, if your poops are hard to pass (constipation), then this might mean that there isn't enough water in your diet or some other underlying issues going on inside your body like low fiber intake or intake of processed foods, etc. Essentially, there are four factors to consider when evaluating your poop.

Four Pooping Signs to Look Out For

Pooping is a crucial part of our everyday life. Just like any bodily function, there are signs that we must look out for to ensure that we maintain a healthy digestive system. Here are some important pooping signs that you should take note of:

Consistency

One of the best ways to determine if your poop is healthy is through its consistency. Your stool should ideally be soft, smooth, and easy to pass. If your poop is hard, dry, or compacted into small balls, you may be constipated. On the other hand, if your poop is loose, watery, and lacks shape, you may be suffering from diarrhea. Both constipation and diarrhea can be caused by poor dietary habits or other underlying medical conditions.

Frequency

The frequency of your bowel movements is another sign that you should keep an eye on. Ideally, you should be excreting once or twice a day. However, this may vary for each person, depending on their age, diet, and lifestyle. If you're not pooping often enough, it could be an indication of constipation. Conversely, if you're pooping too often (more than three times a day), it could signify diarrhea or other digestive issues.

Color

The color of your poop can tell you a lot about your health. In general, poop should be brown due to bilirubin, a byproduct of red blood cell breakdown. If your poop is a different color, it could indicate an underlying medical condition. Red or black stool could signify internal bleeding in the digestive tract. Greenish poop could be because of a high intake of leafy vegetables. Yellow or pale-colored poop could suggest liver or gallbladder problems.

Shape

The shape of your poop may also signal how healthy your poop is. A healthy poop should be sausage-shaped or snake-like, with a smooth surface. If your poop is clumpy, lumpy, or has visible mucus, it could mean constipation, inflammation, or infection in the digestive tract.

In conclusion, paying attention to these pooping signs can help you keep your digestive system healthy. If you notice any abnormal changes in your bowel movements or other digestive symptoms, it's important to seek medical advice. Always remember that a healthy poop means a healthy you!

Seven Types of Poop

When taking the four factors above into consideration, you can experience seven different poops. The Bristol Stool Chart is commonly used by medical professionals to assess the type of stool being passed and provides another clue as to what may be going on internally (DerSarkissian, 2015):

- **Type 1:** Separate hard lumps–This means you might be dehydrated or suffering from constipation due to a low-fiber diet and lack of fruits or veggies in your diet.
- **Type 2:** Sausage-like lumps with cracks on the surface–This could mean you're consuming too much fat and not enough fiber, which causes stools to break down quicker than usual, leading to harder stools that don't move through the digestive system properly.
- **Type 3:** Sausage-shaped lumps but with softness–This means everything is ok and indicates that things are moving along smoothly through the digestive system with no major issues cropping up yet.
- **Type 4:** Smooth and soft snake-like shape–This type typically happens after eating lots of fruits or veggies or taking probiotics for improved gut health, which helps keep stool hydrated and easy to pass without getting stuck inside the digestive tract for long periods of time.
- **Type 5:** Soft blobs with clear-cut edges–If this type appears, then it could indicate a food intolerance or an allergy, so the best way forward would be to eliminate suspect foods from your diet temporarily until symptoms subside, and then reintroduce them one at a

time while monitoring reactions closely each time before adjusting intake accordingly afterward if needed.

- **Type 6:** Fluffy pieces with ragged edges–This can occur when dietary fats are not digested properly due to poor production of bile salts and enzymes needed for digestion. Therefore, reducing fat intake and increasing fiber-rich foods would help improve overall digestion here, too, eventually leading to healthier poops over time once everything gets back into balance again.

- **Type 7:** Watery with no solid pieces–This typically happens after consuming food that irritates the digestive tract or suffering from gastroenteritis. In this case, it is best to drink plenty of fluids and rest while avoiding any spicy or oily foods until symptoms subside before reintroducing them again gradually.

Overall, it's no secret that our poop is an important indicator of overall health and well-being. After all, it can signal potential nutritional deficiencies, food intolerances, dehydration issues, and more. That's why it's so important to get to know your normal poop routine and be able to spot any changes that may indicate an underlying health issue.

The basics boil down to the way you digest food also affects how often you need to go as well as what type of feces are produced in the process. Eating nutrient-dense whole foods helps ensure that your body has all the vitamins and minerals it needs for good digestion and regularity. However, if you eat heavily processed junk food regularly, you may find yourself struggling with constipation due to the lack of fiber in these types of meals. Additionally, staying hydrated is essential for healthy digestion; make sure you're drinking enough water each day.

Understanding your poop can help you stay on top of any potential issues before they become serious and require medical attention. Plus, knowing your normal makes it easier to alert your healthcare provider if anything out of the ordinary pops up. For example, if you're typically a twice-a-day pooper with soft stool consistency, but suddenly everything is dry and hard like rocks, that could signal a dehydration problem or something else going on in your body that needs addressing.

Moreover, paying attention to what comes out the other end is key in identifying gut imbalances such as IBS or small intestinal bacterial overgrowth (SIBO). You may notice extra gas or bloating after eating certain foods, which could indicate food sensitivities, plus diarrhea or constipation due to a disruption in healthy gut bacteria levels. All this information is vital in helping you make informed decisions regarding possible dietary changes or treatments suggested by your healthcare provider.

So next time you take a trip to the bathroom, don't just blindly flush away! Take the time to observe if every-thing looks normal—color and texture should be consistent—then simply jot down any changes you observe on paper or a digital note-taking app like Evernote so you can track any patterns over time. Of course, this doesn't mean obsessing over every little detail but rather being mindful so you can accurately report back to your healthcare provider if needed. Bottom line: keep an eye on those turds!

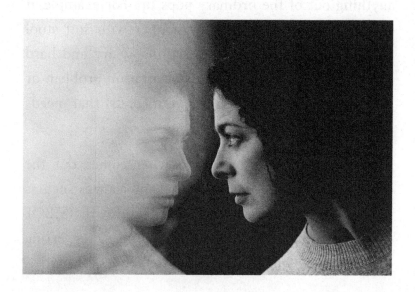

POOPING HABITS AND SCHEDULES—WHAT'S NORMAL?

Now that you know the different poop, it's time to discover which schedule you have and what's normal for you. Pooping habits and schedules can vary from person to person and often depend on diet and lifestyle. Generally speaking, most people have anywhere between one to three bowel movements a day, although some may have more or less than this.

On average, it's normal to poop anywhere from one to three times a day to once every three days. It really depends on the individual and their lifestyle. However, the frequency and consistency of your poop are more vital indicators of your overall health. Therefore, it's more important to pay attention to your body's signals and habits over a long stretch of time. As you become more aware of your body and maybe even track your habits, you can determine what your "normal" is.

It's considered normal for your stools to be soft and easy to pass with no straining or discomfort. If you experience pain, difficulty passing stool, or other concerning symptoms during a bowel movement, it's important to get checked out by a doctor. It could be a sign of something serious such as an infection, IBD, or even cancer.

Overall, everyone has different pooping habits and schedules that work best for them, so don't worry if yours doesn't match up with someone else's—just enjoy being unique!

How to Know and Understand Your Own Body's Natural Pooping Flow

Understanding your own body's natural pooping flow is a great way to ensure that you are staying healthy. There are a few key things you can do to help understand your own body and its digestive habits.

First, you should pay attention to how often you pass a bowel. Paying close attention to how much you typically go could be helpful in understanding your own body's natural flow.

Second, pay close attention to the consistency of your stool. This is because healthy stools contain the right balance of water and fiber, which helps them move quickly through the digestive system. If your stool is hard and dry, this may suggest that you need more fiber in your diet or more water intake throughout the day.

Third, think about what you eat daily as it relates to digestion. Eating balanced meals with plenty of soluble fiber like oats, beans, fruits, and vegetables can help ensure that your food is moving through the digestive system properly so that it doesn't cause constipation or discomfort when passing stools.

Also, consider what times of day you're going to the bathroom, as this could give you insight into your own body's natural schedule. For example, if you typically find yourself pooping in the morning, this could mean that your body is most active during this time of day.

Finally, don't hesitate to reach out for help if you feel something isn't quite right with your pooping habits. Your doctor has lots of experience working with people's bodies, so they will give advice tailored specifically for you based on any further tests they decide might be needed—such as blood work or imaging scans, depending on the situation.

IMPROVING POOPING EXPERIENCES AND HABITS

Improving your pooping experiences and habits can lead to a healthier bowel system and improved overall health. Here are some tips to help improve and maintain healthy pooping habits:

- **Stay hydrated:** Drinking enough water throughout the day can help keep your stool soft and easier to pass. It is recommended to have at least eight glasses of water per day.
- **Eat more fiber:** Fiber is an essential part of a healthy diet, and it can help promote regular bowel movements. Foods such as fruits, vegetables, whole grains, and legumes are excellent sources of fiber.
- **Exercise:** Regular physical activity not only benefits our overall health but also helps to stimulate bowel movements. Maintaining an active lifestyle can help improve the bowel system's functionality.
- **Practice good toilet habits:** Ensure that you are using the toilet fully and not forcing stool out. Also, avoid prolonged sitting and bring a book or phone if necessary.
- **Manage stress:** Stress is a major contributor to digestive issues. Take time to relax and meditate or engage in activities that help reduce stress to prevent constipation and other poop-related problems.
- **Consult a doctor:** If you experience persistent issues such as chronic constipation or diarrhea or are unable to determine a healthy bowel

routine, it's crucial to consult a doctor for evaluation.

Incorporating healthy habits such as staying hydrated, eating a fiber-rich diet, exercising regularly, practicing good toilet habits, and managing stress can help you improve your overall pooping experiences and promote long-term gut health. Remember that everyone's bowel movements differ, so it's essential to determine what works for you and stick to it.

Nine Pooping Tips and Facts for Women

From a young age, we were taught to be more conscious of our bodies and understand the importance of staying healthy. While there might still be people out there who think women don't poop, the fact of the matter is that everyone does.

Here are nine tips and facts about pooping for women to keep in mind:

- The way you sit while pooping is important for your comfort and hygiene. Sitting on the toilet with your knees higher than your hips allows your rectum to relax more and makes elimination easier. This also prevents straining, which can lead to health problems down the line! If you have an extra step stool lying around, give it a shot and see if it makes a difference.

- It's normal to poop after meals, but it's also not a worry if you don't have a bowel movement every time. Everyone's digestive system is different, so it may take some time to regulate your body's rhythms. If your body suddenly changes in its routine and you are not sure why, then you might want to consider what other factors may be involved in your daily routine.

- For women, there is often an increase in pooping during menstruation due to hormonal changes affecting the digestive system. So don't be surprised if you find yourself running to the bathroom more often during that time of the month!

- Caffeine can affect your pooping habits—some people find that after drinking coffee or tea, they experience diarrhea, whereas others notice little difference at all. If you're feeling unsure about how caffeine will affect you, try starting with smaller amounts and see how it goes from there!

- Vacationing or traveling can sometimes lead to constipation due to changes in diet and routine —this is perfectly normal and nothing to worry about as long as constipation doesn't become chronic or severe. Eating plenty of fiber-rich foods such as fruits and vegetables will help keep things moving along nicely!

- Don't ignore the urge to go if you feel like you need to go—pushing it down can cause abdominal discomfort and make elimination more difficult later on when you do go.
- Make sure you stay hydrated—this helps keep everything moving through your system properly and prevents constipation caused by dehydration!
- Pooping should be a relaxing experience—find a comfortable position (such as sitting upright with your feet supported) that helps you relax before going ahead with elimination!
- Don't use laxatives too frequently or without consulting with a doctor first—long-term use of laxatives can lead to dependency and can damage your digestive system over time!

Overall, don't be afraid or feel uncomfortable talking with your doctor if you feel something is off or if you have any questions. They can provide advice tailored specifically for your body based on any results from tests you may take. Taking the time to understand your own body's rhythm and gaining knowledge on proper pooping habits can help ensure everything runs smoothly and healthily.

SUCCESS STORY

According to Linda (2022), Sam had been struggling with IBS for a long time, ever since she had a bout of glandular fever at age 15 that resulted in two mini strokes. A year into her recovery, Sam developed food sensitivities, primarily to gluten and dairy products, which caused her debilitating bloating and pain (Linda, 2022a).

Two years ago, Sam suffered a head injury that resulted in her taking strong medication–including beta blockers—leading to a full flare-up of her IBS symptoms. This included severe bloating, constipation, and even a urinary tract infection, requiring two courses of antibiotics to treat. Her only relief was through using suppositories as well as making lifestyle changes such as reducing stress levels and changing her diet.

However, things began to change for the better after Sam tried an unconventional combination of supplements recommended by a friend and lifestyle changes. Just weeks later, she noticed an incredible improvement in her condition–finally, something that worked.

She felt energized again and was able to begin living life normally once more.

Fast forward one year later, and Sam is still thriving and living symptom-free with IBS. By taking the right combination of probiotics, digestive enzymes, and other gut health supplements regularly, Sam has been able to keep her IBS under control.

Overall, it's been quite a success story for Sam. Her journey is proof that even when faced with chronic conditions such as IBS, taking charge of one's health can lead to amazing results!

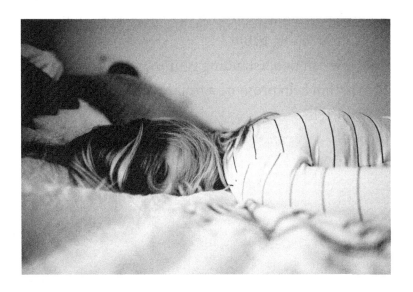

REFLECTION QUESTIONS

- How does your diet affect your pooping habits?
- What are some ways to make sure that you stay regular with your pooping habits?
- Do you already know if you're regular? What's the most common sign of irregularity for you?
- What are some health risks associated with ignoring the urge to go when you need it?
- Have you tried different pooping techniques? How did they work for you?
- What are some benefits you gain from understanding your own individual body and your pooping habits?
- How can understanding your own body's rhythm help promote a healthy lifestyle for yourself?

3

OUR GUTS ARE NOT THE SAME

G ut health is an important topic to understand and maintain, but many people overlook the unique differences between each of our digestive systems. From the bacteria in our stomachs to the enzymes in our intestines, no two guts are exactly alike. That's why having a good sense of your own gut health is so important. It's not just about keeping your stomach feeling great—it's about understanding how your body works and how to keep it strong and healthy.

After all, our gut health affects everything from immunity to inflammation and even mental well-being. With that said, let's inspect the differences in our guts, what makes them unique, and how you can start taking better care of yours too.

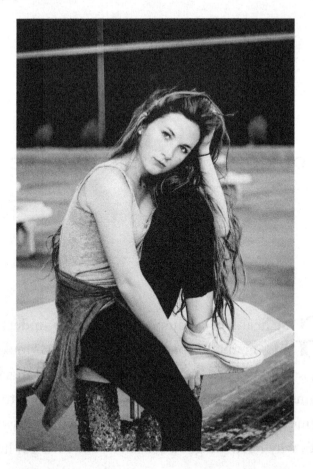

THE PHYSIOLOGICAL DIFFERENCES OF WOMEN

Men and women may seem similar on the surface, but scientifically speaking, they have a myriad of physiological differences. Some of the most significant differences between the two sexes can be found in their digestive systems.

One of the primary physiological differences between men and women is the hormonal balance in their bodies. You may have noticed how our hormones love to cause all sorts of chaos at the most inconvenient times (hello, monthly periods). Well, it turns out that our gut also plays a role in this. Women have higher levels of hormones like estrogen and progesterone. These hormones can affect digestive motility and cause issues like bloating, constipation, and diarrhea. A healthy gut can help maintain hormonal balance and prevent issues like cramps, mood swings, and bloating (Scott, n.d.).

Additionally, women have a more diverse microbiota in their gut than men. This means that they have a wider range of bacteria living in their intestines. While having a diverse microbiota can be beneficial for overall gut health, it can also lead to an imbalance in the gut flora, causing digestive issues (Digestive Health, 2018).

Women also tend to have smaller colons than men. The colon extracts water and electrolytes from waste before it is expelled from the body. The smaller size of the female colon can lead to less efficient absorption of these nutrients, leading to digestive problems (Digestive Health, 2018).

Moreover, women have a slower emptying time, so food takes longer to move through the digestive system.

This can cause constipation or a feeling of fullness and discomfort (Digestive Health, 2018).

Lastly, women produce more bile than men, which can lead to the formation of gallstones. Gallstones are hard, pebble-like deposits that can form in the gallbladder and block the bile duct, causing digestive issues like abdominal pain or nausea (Digestive Health, 2018).

Although physiological differences between genders may cause some GI issues, it doesn't mean these conditions cannot be managed or treated properly by medical professionals. Women should take extra care of themselves if they suspect any of these issues. This can be as simple as changing dietary habits, exercising regularly, relaxing when possible, and visiting their doctor if necessary to ensure quality of life.

The Impact of Gut Health on Women

Let's dive in and explore how women and gut health are related and the common points between them. Women tend to experience more digestive problems, and this can be attributed to several factors.

Did you know that stress can seriously impact women and their gut health? Stress can lead to changes in our gut bacteria, often causing unwanted symptoms such as cramping, bloating, and constipation. So, managing that school, work, or relationship drama is essential for both our mental well-being and our gut health. Make sure you devote some me-time every week to relax and unwind.

Another interesting link between women and gut health is immunity. Believe it or not, 70% of our immune system is located in our gut (EmergenC, n.d.). If we don't take care of it, we're more likely to pick up infections, colds, and other nasties. Getting sick impedes all our daily duties—and nobody has time for that. Thus, ladies, keeping our tummies happy is crucial for staying healthy and rocking that girl power.

Now, let's talk about why gut health is so essential for women. Taking care of our gut can help improve digestion, boost energy levels, and enhance our mood. In fact, around 90% of serotonin, which is considered to be the "happy hormone," is produced in our gut (Barker, n.d.). So, if we neglect our gut health, we are more likely to be grumpy and fatigued.

Women who don't care for their gut health might experience a bunch of unpleasant consequences. Aside from problems with using the bathroom and digestion, an unhappy gut has been linked to skin issues (hello, acne) and a higher risk of developing chronic diseases such as obesity, diabetes, and heart disease later in life (Steber, 2018).

In a nutshell, taking care of our gut health as women is essential for our overall well-being. It helps maintain hormonal balance, boosts our mood, strengthens our immune system, and prevents many health issues. So, let's embrace the power of a healthy gut and rock our amazing, strong, and beautiful selves.

STRESS AND FEMALE HORMONES: A DELICATE BALANCE IN WOMEN'S HEALTH

Our bodies are a complex and interconnected system, with each part playing a significant role in our overall well-being. One of the most fascinating relationships in our body is the connection between stress, hormones, and the gut, particularly for women. This intricate dance between the brain, the endocrine system, and the digestive system can have both short-term and long-term effects on our health. Let's explore this connection and see just how these factors influence one another.

Stress and the Stress Hormones

Stress, the body's natural response to threats or challenges, can come in various forms. We can experience stress through physical, emotional, or psychological sensations. When we're stressed, the brain triggers stress hormones, like cortisol and adrenaline, to prepare our body to take action. These hormones help us by increasing heart rate, diverting blood flow to essential organs, and elevating glucose levels, which can cause inflammation in the gut, leading to a variety of digestive problems, such as IBS.

While short-term stress can be helpful, chronic stress can lead to an imbalance in hormone levels over time, causing health issues. For women, these imbalances can affect reproductive health, menstruation, and even menopause.

Hormones and Women's Health

Women's bodies experience fluctuations in hormone levels throughout their lives, particularly during menstrual cycles, pregnancy, and menopause. These hormonal changes can impact mood, energy levels, and overall well-being.

For instance, during menstruation or premenstrual syndrome (PMS), women may experience symptoms like irritability, depression, and fatigue due to hormonal imbalances. Similarly, during menopause, estrogen and progesterone levels decline, leading to symptoms like hot flashes, mood swings, and sleep disturbances (Steber, 2018).

These hormones can also affect our gut and digestive health. For instance, when estrogen and progesterone levels are low, the GI tract is more vulnerable to inflammatory responses, which can lead to GI issues like IBS.

Our hormone levels can be influenced by various factors, including stress, diet, exercise, and environmental factors. Therefore, it's crucial for women to maintain a healthy lifestyle to minimize hormonal imbalances.

Pregnancy, Hormones, and Gut Health

Pregnancy is a beautiful and exciting chapter in a woman's life. However, it can also come along with some challenges. One of these challenges might be digestive issues. During pregnancy, hormonal changes occur that can affect a woman's gut health, leading to discomfort and other digestive problems.

Hormones like progesterone and estrogen play a vital role in pregnancy. Progesterone, for example, is responsible for relaxing the muscles in the uterus to prepare for the baby's growth. However, it also relaxes muscles in the digestive tract, causing food to move more slowly through the intestines. This can result in constipation, bloating, and gas.

Estrogen, on the other hand, increases blood flow to the uterus and placenta, supporting the baby's growth. However, it can also cause the lining of the digestive tract to thicken, which can hinder nutrient absorption and cause inflammation. Additionally, during pregnancy, the gut microbiome undergoes changes due to hormonal fluctuations, making a woman more susceptible to GI infections.

Therefore, it is crucial for pregnant women to take care of their gut health. This includes consuming a diet rich in fiber, staying hydrated, and engaging in physical activities that promote proper digestion. Women may also consider probiotic supplements to promote a better balance.

In the end, pregnancy can have a significant impact on a woman's gut health due to hormonal changes. Therefore, it is essential to take precautionary measures to ensure optimal digestive health during this exciting time. By being attentive to diet, hydration, exercise, and probiotic supplements, women can support their gut microbiome and enjoy a successful, healthy pregnancy.

The Gut Connection

Emerging research has shown that the gut and the brain are connected through the gut-brain axis (Cryan et al., 2019). This complex communication system allows our gut to send signals to the brain and vice versa. This means that stress and hormonal imbalances can impact the gut microbiome, leading to issues like IBS, bloating, and inflammation.

The connection between internal and external factors in the gut is particularly important for women due to their unique hormonal fluctuations. Chronic stress and imbalances in hormone levels can critically impair gut health, further exacerbating health concerns.

Promoting a Healthy Balance

Understanding the connection our gut has with the rest of our body is the first step to achieving balanced health. Women should focus on managing stress levels, maintaining a healthy diet, exercising regularly, and prioritizing self-care. Incorporating probiotics or prebiotics to support a healthy gut microbiome can also be beneficial. By nurturing this delicate balance between our mind, body, and gut, we can improve our overall well-being and navigate life's challenges with greater resilience.

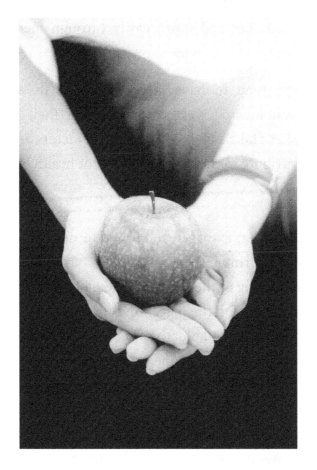

MEN AND GUT HEALTH: A CLOSER LOOK AT THE DIGESTIVE DIFFERENCES

In general, it is believed that men tend to have fewer digestive concerns compared to women. The reasons behind this apparent difference are both interesting and diverse, encompassing hormonal, physiological, and lifestyle factors. For example, food can pass through quicker and more easily through men since their stomachs have faster emptying times.

They also tend to have larger colons than women, which can mean fewer toxins entering their bloodstream. Let's take a closer look at these factors and how they contribute to the differences in gut health between the sexes.

- **Hormones:** Estrogen and progesterone, two female hormones, have a direct impact on the functioning of the GI tract. These hormones can slow down the digestion process, leading to constipation and bloating. On the other hand, men's primary hormone, testosterone, does not have the same effect on gut motility. Thus, men tend to experience fewer digestive issues related to hormonal fluctuations.
- **Menstrual cycle:** A woman's menstrual cycle adds an extra dimension to the gender differences in gut health. According to research, the hormone fluctuations during the cycle impact gut function, making women more susceptible to digestive problems like bloating, constipation, and diarrhea.
- **Anatomical differences:** The female reproductive system occupies a more significant portion of the pelvic cavity, leaving

less space for other organs, including the colon. This spatial limitation can lead to a slower transit time for waste elimination in women, increasing the likelihood of constipation and related issues.

- **Muscle mass and metabolism:** Men typically have a higher percentage of muscle mass than women, which has been linked to a faster metabolism. Consequently, food moves through the digestive system more quickly in men, reducing the chances of constipation or bloating.

- **Lifestyle factors:** There is some evidence that men are more likely to engage in physical activities, which can contribute to better gut health. Exercise has been proven to help improve the digestive system by promoting regular bowel movements and preventing constipation.

Although both genders share some similarities when it comes to digestion, there are several physiological differences that make women more likely to experience certain GI issues than men. It is important that women understand these differences so they can take preventative measures and seek medical assistance if necessary. With the right knowledge and self-care strategies, women can stay healthy and keep their GI systems functioning at their best.

In the end, like their female counterparts, men are not immune to digestive issues. Common GI problems in men include constipation, indigestion, heartburn, IBS, and gallstones. While being male certainly doesn't exempt them from experiencing digestive issues, women tend to have more digestive problems and more severe symptoms than men.

GI TESTING

GI disorders can be tricky to diagnose because a lot of them have overlapping symptoms. For example, IBS and Crohn's Disease can both cause abdominal pain, diarrhea, and weight loss. But fear not; even though it may seem impossible to tell them apart, there are tests that can help give you the answer you need.

Ultrasounds, computed tomography (CT), and magnetic resonance imaging (MRI) are all imaging techniques used to create pictures of the abdomen that help doctors detect various GI disorders. A barium swallow or upper GI series is another test used to examine the esophagus, stomach, and small intestine by having the patient drink a chalky liquid called barium so it shows up on an X-ray.

An upper GI endoscopy is when a doctor puts a thin tube in your mouth down your throat so they can get an up-close view of your esophagus, stomach, and small intestine. A barium enema is similar to a barium swallow, but it looks for abnormalities in the large intestine or colon instead. Sigmoidoscopy and colonoscopy are two tests where doctors put flexible tubes with cameras into your rectum so they can look at the entire inside of the large intestine for any signs of disease.

So if you've been experiencing ongoing GI issues, don't worry. There's still hope in finding out what's going on. It might take some tests here and there, but eventually, you'll get an answer to what's causing your discomfort —even if it means wearing a bright blue gown during your ultrasound.

Chronic GI

GI issues can be a real nuisance, but when they're chronic, this can indicate a much deeper problem. Irritable bowel disease is an umbrella term for diseases that cause inflammation and irritation of the digestive tract, including ulcerative colitis and Crohn's disease. If left untreated, these diseases can lead to serious health complications such as malnutrition or ulcers in the large intestine. IBS is another common chronic GI issue that causes cramps, bloating, and changes in bowel habits, such as diarrhea or constipation.

The exact cause of IBS is unknown. However, it may be linked to stress and poor diet. Gallstones are hardened deposits of digestive fluid that form in the gallbladder, which can also cause abdominal pain, nausea, and vomiting if they become lodged in the bile ducts. Colon cancer is another potentially serious issue caused by uncontrolled cell growth within the colon or rectum, which could lead to bleeding or blockages within the intestine.

Gastritis refers to inflammation of the stomach lining caused by infection with bacteria such as H. pylori or long-term use of NSAIDS like ibuprofen, which can lead to stomach pain, indigestion, bloating, and nausea if left untreated. Lastly, esophagitis is an inflammation of the esophagus that occurs when acid from your stomach backs up into your throat causing heartburn and difficulty swallowing food.

It's important to pay attention to any chronic GI signs you may have as they could point toward deeper issues; having them checked out sooner rather than later will help you avoid more serious health problems down the road, so don't delay! Sometimes, dietary changes or medications may help manage symptoms, but always check with your doctor first before beginning any new treatments.

COMMON DIGESTIVE ISSUES FOR WOMEN

Digestive health is an essential aspect of overall well-being. However, women are more likely to experience certain digestive issues because of factors such as hormonal imbalances, dietary habits, and stress. In this guide, we'll explore some common digestive problems that affect women, along with helpful tips and insights about diagnosis, treatment, and prevention.

Irritable Bowel Syndrome

IBS is a common GI disorder characterized by chronic abdominal pain, bloating, and alternating bouts of constipation and diarrhea (Ensley, 2007). It affects roughly 10–15% of the population, and women are twice as likely to experience IBS symptoms as men (Ensley, 2007). Researchers believe the female hormonal fluctuations throughout the menstrual cycle may contribute to the increased prevalence in women.

Tips: Keeping a food diary can help identify trigger foods, and incorporating stress-relieving activities like yoga or meditation can provide relief. Doctors may also recommend a low Fermentable Oligo-, Di-, and

Monosaccharides and Polyols (FODMAP) diet, which reduces foods that can provoke IBS symptoms. This diet includes avoiding certain high-fructose fruits and vegetables like apples, onions, pears, watermelon, artichokes, and mushrooms.

Gastroesophageal Reflux Disease

Gastroesophageal reflux disease (GERD) is a condition where stomach acid frequently flows back into the esophagus, leading to heartburn, regurgitation, and difficulty swallowing (Mayo Clinic, 2020). Fluctuating hormones throughout the menstrual cycle, as well as during pregnancy, can affect the lower esophageal sphincter (LES), leading to a higher risk of GERD among women.

Tips: Eating smaller meals, avoiding fatty or spicy foods, and staying upright after eating can help manage GERD. Over-the-counter antacids and proton pump inhibitors are also available for those suffering more frequently or severely.

Inflammatory Bowel Disease

IBD, which includes Crohn's disease and ulcerative colitis, is characterized by inflammation in the digestive tract (Ensley, 2007). Women with IBD may experience additional symptoms related to menstruation and hormonal changes, such as worsening IBD symptoms premenstrually.

Tips: Treatment for IBD often involves medication to reduce inflammation, and sometimes, surgery may be necessary. Maintaining a healthy diet and staying in close contact with a healthcare provider can be beneficial in managing IBD effectively.

Gallstones

Gallstones form when substances in bile, such as cholesterol or bilirubin, harden in the gallbladder (Ensley, 2007). Women are at a higher risk of developing gallstones than men, mainly due to hormonal changes during pregnancy or as a side effect of birth control pills. Symptoms may include sudden and severe abdominal pain, fever, and jaundice.

Tips: A low-fat diet and keeping a healthy weight can help prevent gallstones. Treatment may involve medications or surgery to remove the gallbladder if the pain becomes frequent or severe.

Celiac Disease

Celiac disease is an autoimmune disorder where your body reacts negatively to gluten, a protein found in wheat, barley, and rye (Mayo Clinic, 2021). This reaction causes inflammation and damage to the small intestine lining, leading to malabsorption of nutrients. Women with celiac disease may experience irregular periods, fertility issues, and osteoporosis because of malabsorption of nutrients.

Tips: The only treatment for celiac disease is a strict gluten-free diet, which allows the small intestine to heal and prevents further damage. Consulting a dietitian can be helpful in adapting to a gluten-free lifestyle.

Constipation

Constipation is a common digestive issue for women, especially during pregnancy. It occurs when your bowels are unable to move food through the intestines properly. Symptoms of constipation can include infrequent or difficult-to-pass stools and feeling bloated or uncomfortable after meals.

Tips: Eating high-fiber foods such as fruits, vegetables, and whole grains can help keep your bowels moving.

Drinking plenty of water and exercising regularly can also help ease constipation. If these measures are not helping, speak with your doctor about taking a laxative or other medications for relief.

Small Intestine Bacteria Growth

SIBO is a condition where bacteria populate the small intestine in higher numbers than normal. This can lead to abdominal pain, bloating, nausea, and diarrhea. Women are more likely to have SIBO due to contraceptives and other hormones that affect gut motility, making them more susceptible to infection.

Tips: Avoiding processed foods and added sugars, as well as increasing intake of probiotics, can help reduce symptoms. If necessary, antibiotics may be prescribed to kill off the overgrown bacteria population.

Heartburn

Heartburn is a burning sensation that occurs when stomach acid moves up into the esophagus. It can be caused by eating spicy or acidic foods, drinking alcohol, or lying down after a meal. Women are more likely to experience heartburn during pregnancy because of hormonal changes and increased pressure on the stomach by the fetus.

Tips: Avoiding triggers such as certain foods and drinks can help prevent heartburn. Eating smaller meals and avoiding lying down after eating can also help. Over-the-counter antacids or medications such as proton pump inhibitors can provide relief if needed. Speak to your doctor about which treatment is best for you.

Colon Cancer

Colon cancer occurs when abnormal cells grow in the large intestine. Women who are over the age of 50, have a family history of colon cancer, or lead an inactive life-style are at an increased risk for this condition. Symptoms may include changes in bowel habits, blood in the stool, abdominal pain, and fatigue.

Tips: Regular screening for colon cancer is recommended for those at an increased risk; this usually involves a colonoscopy. Adopting a healthy diet, including regular exercise, and avoiding tobacco can also lower the risk of developing colon cancer. Speak with your doctor about which screening method is most appropriate for you.

Gastroparesis

Gastroparesis is a digestive disorder where the stomach takes too long to empty its contents into the small intestine. It can cause nausea, vomiting, bloating, and other GI symptoms. Women are more likely to develop gastroparesis, especially those with diabetes or prior abdominal surgery.

Tips: Dietary changes such as eating smaller meals more frequently and avoiding fatty or fibrous foods can help manage symptoms. Taking medications such as metoclopramide may also be prescribed to help the stomach empty more quickly. If lifestyle modifications do not provide adequate relief, surgery may be necessary.

Leaky Gut Syndrome

Leaky gut syndrome is a condition where the lining of the intestines becomes damaged, allowing bacteria and toxins to leak into the bloodstream. Symptoms may include abdominal pain, bloating, fatigue, and food sensitivities. Women are more likely than men to have this condition due to hormones that affect intestinal permeability.

Tips: Following an anti-inflammatory diet can help reduce inflammation in the intestines and improve symptoms. Probiotics and digestive enzymes may also be beneficial in restoring gut health.

While women are prone to various digestive issues, understanding the root causes and seeking appropriate medical assistance can significantly help manage and prevent these conditions. Maintaining a balanced diet, practicing stress management, and staying informed about your digestive health can lead to a happier and healthier you!

SUCCESS STORY

Rebecca, a determined and fitness-conscious woman, started experiencing a myriad of health issues that left her feeling helpless and unrecognizable. However, driven by perseverance, she found her way back to a healthy life through a three-step system that focused on healing and restoring her health, ultimately leading her to feel better than ever. Her story is a testament to the fact that with dedication and the right approach, one can successfully overcome their most daunting health challenges (Mulhall, 2021).

Rebecca's health troubles began as a combination of severe fatigue, bloating, short-term memory loss, confusion, and severe swelling. As she continued training harder and reducing her calorie intake, her muscles seemed to vanish, replaced by unwanted fat. She experienced a decrease in her metabolic rate, an increase in androgens, and an excessive overproduction of dopamine—all these factors were closely interlinked, making it complex to identify and treat her condition.

Taking control of her situation, Rebecca turned to a three-step system that improved her symptoms and ultimately led to her successful recovery. The steps included identifying the root cause, balancing hormones and stress levels, and rebuilding her metabolism.

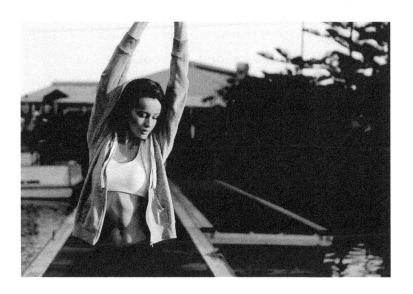

Through a combination of understanding her body's unique needs, focusing on rebalancing her hormones, and restoring her metabolism, Rebecca was able to regain control of her life and her health. In time, her symptoms faded, her health returned, and she began to thrive once more. By sharing her journey of healing and recovery, Rebecca now serves as an inspiration to others struggling with similar health challenges, giving them hope that they, too, can find a path back to health and happiness.

REFLECTION QUESTIONS

- Do you have any common digestive issues?
- What methods have you used to manage any digestive issues that you have?
- How does understanding the root causes of common digestive issues among women help you better manage your own health?
- In what other ways can you see how your gut health affects your overall health and well-being?
- What are some simple changes that you can make to your diet or lifestyle in order to promote better gut health?

PAUSE FOR THOUGHT

"Health is the greatest of human blessings."

— HIPPOCRATES

Why did you pick up this book?

I'd hazard a guess that it's because you've been experiencing digestive symptoms and looking into how you can handle them yourself without needing to discuss them with a medical practitioner – or anyone else for that matter!

As we said in the introduction, this isn't something we like to talk about, particularly as women. We struggle on alone, often brushing our symptoms under the carpet and assuming it must be normal to feel this way.

It's normal only in that so many people live with it – but it's not inevitable, and as you're discovering, it's entirely possible to make the changes necessary to get your gut health back under control.

I'm passionate about giving as many people the tools they need to do this as I can – because I know how many people suffer in silence, and I want to empower them to take control, even if they can't bring themselves to talk about what they're experiencing. And I'd like to ask for your help.

Don't worry – there's a quick and easy way for you to do that, and you don't need to share your own story unless you really want to.

By leaving a review of this book on Amazon, you'll show other people struggling with digestive symptoms where they can find the guidance they need to get their health back on track.

Simply by letting new readers know how this book has helped you and what they'll find inside, you'll point them in the direction of all the information and guidance they need to take control of their gut health.

Thank you so much for your support. When it comes to conditions we rarely talk about in society, spreading the word is the most valuable thing we can do.

4

GUT HEALTH AND OUR PHYSICAL AND MENTAL WELL-BEING

S o, why is gut health so important for women, you may wonder? Allow me to take you through the ins and outs of this fascinating topic, and by the end of our journey, you'll understand why tending to your gut is essential for a harmonious, healthy life.

At the very core of maintaining excellent gut health is our microbiome—a bustling community of trillions of microorganisms residing in our GI tract. As we reviewed, these tiny tenants are responsible for a myriad of critical functions in our bodies, such as digesting food, producing essential vitamins, regulating metabolism, and even supporting our immune system. Equipped with this knowledge, it's evident that ensuring a thriving and balanced gut flora should be one of our top priorities!

Interestingly, studies have shown that women's gut health has a unique connection to their hormonal balance (Scott, n.d.). For instance, fluctuations in estrogen levels during menstruation, pregnancy, and menopause can significantly impact our gut's microbial composition. In return, a poorly balanced gut can cause undesirable effects on our hormonal balance, leading to conditions such as polycystic ovary syndrome (PCOS) and endometriosis.

It's also essential to acknowledge that IBS, a disorder that causes altered bowel habits and leads to abdominal pain, predominantly affects women. Research has discovered that women suffering from IBS frequently experience anxiety and depression, further emphasizing the importance of nurturing our gut health (Scott, n.d.).

At first glance, these conditions may not seem connected, but that's far from the truth. By giving our gut health the attention and care it deserves, we can ensure that our bodies and minds remain in optimal condition—and ultimately, embrace a life full of vitality and joy.

THE MICROBIOTA-GUT-BRAIN AXIS: A FASCINATING CONNECTION EXPLAINED

Have you ever heard the saying, "trust your gut?" Well, it turns out there's more science behind the idea that our gut and brain are connected. One of the most exciting discoveries in recent years is the microbiota-gut-brain axis, which refers to the complex communication network between our gut microbiota, digestive system, and brain. To put it simply, it's a conversation happening between the little critters in our gut and our brain that impacts our overall health and well-being. Let's dive a bit deeper into this fascinating connection and how it works.

The connection between our microbiota and brain is a two-way street, with messages being sent back and forth via several routes, including the nervous system, immune system, and hormones. Communication between the gut and brain is mainly controlled by the vagus nerve, which joins the brainstem to the abdomen. The vagus nerve allows the brain and gut to send messages to each other about the state of the body, what nutrients we require, and any potential threats.

One of the key components of this communication system is the production of neurotransmitters by our gut microbiota. Neurotransmitters are chemical messengers that transmit signals between nerve cells in our brains (Cleveland Clinic, 2022). You may have heard of some of them, like serotonin, dopamine, and gamma-aminobutyric acid (GABA), which are involved in regulating our mood, appetite, sleep, and stress response. Astonishingly, about 90% of our body's serotonin and 50% of our dopamine are produced in the gut, suggesting a strong link between gut microbiota and brain function (Scott, n.d.).

Another key component is the production of metabolites. Metabolites are a byproduct of the digestive process, such as short-chain fatty acids, which plays a role in brain health. By influencing the release of hormones and neurotransmitters, these metabolites can have a direct impact on our mood and mental well-being. This fascinating connection is known as the microbiota-gut-brain axis, and it highlights just how powerful our gut health is for our overall well-being.

So, what does all this mean for our health and well-being? Studies have shown that disruptions to the microbiota-gut-brain axis can cause a range of mental health issues, including anxiety, depression, and even neurodegenerative diseases like Alzheimer's and Parkinson's (Cryan et al., 2019). Moreover, imbalances in gut microbiota, also known as dysbiosis, have been associated with chronic inflammation, obesity, and metabolic disorders. This highlights the importance of maintaining a healthy and diverse gut microbiome for our overall health.

Overall, the microbiota-gut-brain axis is an extraordinary communication system that's critical to our overall health and well-being. By understanding and nurturing this connection, we can take actionable steps to improve our mental and physical health. So the next time you "trust your gut," know that there's a fantastic world of microscopic creatures in there, working tirelessly to keep you feeling balanced and healthy.

Vagus Nerve, Enteric Nervous System, and Central Nervous System

The vagus nerve is an important communication pathway that connects the enteric nervous system (ENS) and the central nervous system (CNS). The CNS sends signals down to the ENS, which then controls digestion, secretions, and motor responses of the GI tract. Similarly, when the ENS detects changes in food composition or environment, it sends information back up to the CNS in order to regulate further response.

Interestingly, recent research has shown that the microbiome, the collection of microorganisms living in our gut, plays a crucial role in the relationship between the vagus nerve, ENS, and CNS. The microbiome produces chemicals that communicate with the vagus nerve, which in turn signals the CNS, leading to changes in our physical and mental health.

One important way in which the microbiome affects our health is through its impact on inflammation. Chronic inflammation has been linked to many diseases, including depression, anxiety, autoimmune diseases, and cancer. The microbiome produces short-chain fatty acids that have anti-inflammatory properties and play a vital role in keeping inflammation in check.

The microbiome also affects our mood and behavior by producing neurotransmitters such as serotonin and dopamine. Most serotonin is in the gut, and about 50% of dopamine is too. Studies have shown that changes in the microbiome can lead to alterations in mood, behavior, and even social interactions (Cryan et al., 2019).

Another concern is the disruption of the gut-brain axis, which links the ENS and CNS. Disruption of this axis can lead to a wide range of physical and mental illnesses. For example, studies have shown that IBS is associated with an imbalance in the microbiome. By restoring balance in the gut, many IBS patients have seen improvements in their symptoms.

The importance of maintaining a healthy gut micro-biome cannot be overstated. Eating a diet rich in fiber, fermented foods, prebiotics, and probiotics can help promote a healthy microbiome, which in turn can benefit our physical and mental health. Additionally, reducing stress, getting plenty of sleep, and avoiding unnecessary antibiotic use can all have a positive impact on the microbiome and ultimately support our overall well-being.

As you can see, the vagus nerve, ENS, CNS, and the microbiome all have a complex and interconnected relationship that significantly impacts our physical and mental health. By understanding the role of each of these systems, we can take steps to maintain a healthy microbiome and support optimal physical and mental health.

The Gut and Your Physical Health

Recent research has shed light on the significant impact that the gut has on both our physical and mental health. In this section, we will explore the amazing world of our gut and help you understand its vital role in keeping us healthy and happy.

First things first—let's explore how the gut affects our physical health. Our GI tract is home to trillions of microorganisms. These tiny organisms play a pivotal role in not just our digestion but also in regulating many aspects of our health, including our immune system, metabolism, and even our ability to fight off infections. Having a diverse and balanced gut microbiota is essential for maintaining good physical health.

Research has shown that poor gut health can lead to a range of physical issues. For example, a compromised gut can lead to digestive problems such as bloating, constipation, and diarrhea. Furthermore, studies have linked poor gut health to other health conditions, such as allergies, autoimmune disorders, and mental health issues (Cryan et al., 2019).

One sign that our gut health is affecting us physically is frequent stomach issues. If you experience consistent bloating, cramps, or discomfort after eating, it could be a sign of an underlying gut problem. Additionally, skin issues such as acne and eczema can also be linked to gut health. Another sign is a weakened immune system. This can result in frequent infections or illnesses.

To maintain good gut health, it is important to have a balanced diet rich in fiber, whole foods, and probiotics. Reducing stress can also improve the gut and its symptoms. If you are experiencing persistent physical symptoms, it is important to consult with a medical professional to identify any underlying gut issues.

In conclusion, maintaining good gut health is essential for physical well-being. Being aware of the signs and symptoms of gut issues can help identify and address any underlying problems. By prioritizing good gut health through a healthy diet and lifestyle, we can establish and maintain a healthier body overall.

The Gut and Your Mental Health

Now let's delve into the fascinating connection between our gut and mental health. The significance of women's gut health extends beyond physical well-being and into the realm of mental health. The gut has earned the nickname "the second brain" for good reason—it contains a vast network of neurons that are in constant communication with our brain. This gut-brain axis allows our gut microbiota to influence our mood, anxiety levels, and overall mental well-being. As we mentioned, one of the key players in this communication is serotonin, a neurotransmitter that regulates many of our habits, which is mainly produced in the gut.

An imbalance in our gut microbiota can lead to changes in our brain's neurochemistry, which may trigger anxiety, depression, or other mental health issues. Recent studies have shown that certain strains of gut bacteria can produce substances that hold the potential to reduce anxiety and depression and even improve memory and cognitive function (Cryan et al., 2019).

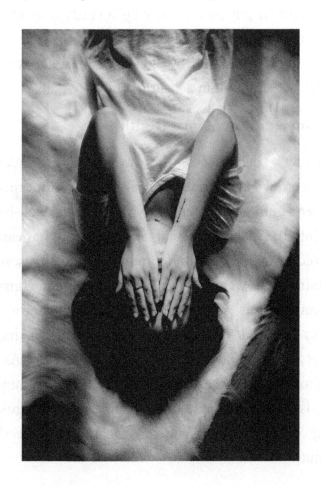

TYPES OF BACTERIA FOUND IN THE GUT AND WHAT THEY MEAN

When most people hear the word "bacteria," they likely think of infections and illnesses. However, not all bacteria are bad. In fact, as we mention, the vast majority of bacteria living in our guts are harmless or even beneficial.

Commensal Bacteria

There are many types of commensal bacteria that coexist harmlessly with us. These bacteria provide a variety of benefits, such as aiding in digestion, producing vitamins, and even training our immune systems to distinguish between "good" and "bad" bacteria. Other types of bacteria found in the gut microbiome include Bacteroidetes, which are beneficial bacteria that help to digest food and keep the intestines healthy. Here, we will discuss some of the most common types of bacteria in your digestive tract and why they are important.

Firmicutes

Firmicutes are the most abundant bacteria in the gut, making up about 50% of the total bacteria (Rinninella et al., 2019). They are responsible for breaking down complex carbohydrates and converting them into energy. They also play a role in the absorption of nutrients and the regulation of inflammation. If the Firmicutes levels are too high, it can lead to obesity, while low levels may increase the risk for IBD.

Bacteroidetes

Bacteroidetes are important for breaking down complex sugars and producing short-chain fatty acids, which are essential for maintaining a healthy gut lining (Rinninella et al., 2019). They also help to regulate inflammation and the immune system. Imbalances in Bacteroidetes levels have been linked to several diseases, including obesity, diabetes, and IBD.

Actinobacteria

Actinobacteria help to break down complex carbohydrates and produce vitamin K (Rinninella et al., 2019). They are also involved in the production of antimicrobial compounds that protect against pathogenic bacteria. Low levels of actinobacteria have been associated with IBD and allergies.

Proteobacteria

Proteobacteria are diverse and include both beneficial and pathogenic species (Rinninella et al., 2019). They are involved in the breakdown of amino acids and the production of nitrogen. Out-of-balance levels of proteobacteria have been linked to various gut disorders like ulcerative colitis, Crohn's disease, and IBS.

Fusobacteria

Fusobacteria are a small portion of the gut microbiome and have been linked to ulcerative colitis and colon cancer (Rinninella et al., 2019). It comes from the same family as proteobacteria but is less commonly found in healthy individuals.

Verrucomicrobia

Verrucomicrobia play a key role in regulating the mucous layer of the gut, which is essential for protecting the gut lining from harmful pathogens. Additionally, they help maintain gut health and reduce inflammation levels. Low levels of Verrucomicrobia have been linked to metabolic disorders.

Lactobacillus

This is a genus of bacteria that aids in digestion. They help break down carbohydrates and produce lactic acid. Doing so prevents the growth of harmful bacteria in our guts. Studies have also found that some strains of Lactobacillus can reduce inflammation, boost the immune system, and even aid in weight management (Rinninella et al., 2019).

Bifidobacteria

These bacteria are another beneficial genus that improves our gut health. It aids in digestion and helps to protect us from pathogenic bacteria. Studies have found that Bifidobacteria can help reduce inflammation and boost the immune system (Rinninella et al., 2019).

Overall, the balance of different types of bacteria in the gut is crucial for maintaining good health. Any imbalance in the gut microbiome—whether healthy or unhealthy originally—can lead to various gut issues like diarrhea, bloating, gas, constipation, and even neurological disorders like depression and anxiety. Therefore, your gut health is essential for your overall well-being, and choosing a healthy diet supporting beneficial bacteria in the gut will have positive outcomes for your health as a whole.

Clostridium Difficile

Now that we understand some of the positive bacteria in our gut, let's review some of the unhealthy bacteria that can affect our gut well-being. One of the most well-known harmful bacteria is Clostridium difficile. This bacterium can cause infections that range from mild diarrhea to life-threatening inflammation of the colon.

Clostridium difficile is important because it can cause a range of infections, from mild diarrhea to inflammation. These infections are usually caused by an overgrowth of bad bacteria, which can happen when the good bacteria in the gut are out of balance, usually as a result of taking antibiotics.

When bad bacteria like Clostridium difficile are out of balance in the gut, they can cause inflammation and damage to the lining of the gut, leading to diarrhea, stomach pain, and other unpleasant symptoms. In severe cases, the infection can cause severe inflammation of the colon, which can be life-threatening.

Clostridium difficile is broken into three categories: non-severe, severe, and fulminant. Non-severe cases can be treated with antibiotics, while more serious cases may require hospitalization for supportive care and IV antibiotics. Some examples of non-severe Clostridium difficile infections include diarrhea, abdominal pain, and fever. Severe cases are more serious and can lead to complications such as pseudomembranous colitis, toxic megacolon, and sepsis. Fulminant cases are the most severe and may require surgery to remove part of the colon or even a complete colectomy.

The key to preventing or managing Clostridium difficile infections is to keep your gut flora balanced by maintaining a healthy diet, taking probiotics, and avoiding unnecessary use of antibiotics. If you do happen to get a Clostridium difficile infection, it's important to get it treated right away.

When the balance of bacteria in the gut microbiome is disrupted, it can lead to health issues. An overgrowth of harmful bacteria like Clostridium difficile can cause infections, while a lack of commensal bacteria can lead to problems like inflammation and autoimmune disorders.

In the end, while there are certainly harmful types of bacteria that can be present in the gut microbiome, most bacteria are harmless or even beneficial. By understanding the different bacteria and how they can impact our health, we can ensure we maintain a healthy balance of bacteria in our gut.

SIGNS AND SYMPTOMS OF AN UNHEALTHY GUT

Your gut and microbiome are crucial to your overall health and wellness. They are responsible for digesting the food you eat, absorbing vital nutrients, and keeping harmful bacteria at bay. However, if your gut is unhealthy, it can lead to several uncomfortable and sometimes painful symptoms.

One of the most common signs of an unhealthy gut is constipation or diarrhea. This can lead to feelings of discomfort and bloating in the stomach, along with cramping or pain in the abdomen. Acid reflux and nausea are also common symptoms, making it difficult to enjoy meals or maintain an appetite.

Other symptoms of an unhealthy gut can include unexplained weight loss or gain, fatigue, and changes in mood or energy levels. You may experience skin problems, such as rashes and acne, or have trouble sleeping at night. One of the more embarrassing symptoms of an unhealthy gut is bad breath or a coated tongue, along with being gassy and bloated.

Overall, these signs may indicate an imbalance within the gut microbiome or possible infection, such as SIBO. If you're concerned, reach out to a professional for a more in-depth evaluation. A dedicated professional can help you identify the root cause of your gut problems and provide you with the necessary treatment to ease your symptoms.

In addition to medical treatment, there are several lifestyle changes you can make to promote a healthier gut. In the end, good gut health care is essential for your overall well-being. By understanding the signs and symptoms of an unhealthy gut, you can take proactive steps to maintain optimal gut health and enjoy a happier, healthier life.

Uncommon Symptoms to Look Out For

Aside from the more common signs mentioned above, there are a few other potential indications of an unhealthy gut that may not be so obvious. These might include joint aches and pains, white patches on the tongue known as oral thrush (this is caused by a yeast overgrowth), or recurring headaches and migraines.

If you're experiencing any unusual digestive symptoms that don't fit with your normal routine, it's important to pay attention. Women, in particular, should know the following signs and symptoms that could show more serious issues and require immediate medical attention. For example, if you find yourself experiencing black or tarry stools, this can show bleeding in your upper GI tract, likely due to an ulcer or polyps in the stomach or small intestine. If left untreated and ignored, these concerns can get worse quickly!

Vomiting blood is also a sign of a GI issue which should be discussed with a doctor right away. Unusual abdominal pain can also point to a problem—particularly if it's located on just one side of your body, as this could signal an obstruction such as appendicitis or ovarian cysts. Also, if you've been having any rectal bleeding—especially accompanied by severe abdominal pain—there's a chance you may have an intestinal infection that requires immediate medical attention. So keep an eye out for any strange digestive symptoms and contact your doctor if something doesn't feel quite right.

Poor concentration and memory can also be related to an unbalanced gut flora. Other unusual symptoms could include food sensitivities or allergies, even if you have never had them before. This can happen when your body is no longer able to properly digest certain foods due to a lack of beneficial bacteria within the gut.

Improving Central Nervous System, Enteric Nervous System, and the Vagus Nerve

To optimize this connection, there are several methods that can be implemented.

Firstly, maintaining a healthy and varied diet is key to promoting a healthy microbiome. Consuming a diet rich in fiber, fermented foods, and prebiotics can help support the growth of beneficial gut bacteria. Conversely, a diet high in processed foods and sugar can negatively impact the microbiome and disrupt the gut-brain connection.

Physical activity is another important aspect of improving the connection between the nervous system and microbiome. Exercise has been shown to increase the diversity and abundance of beneficial gut bacteria, as well as improve communication between the gut and brain.

Additionally, stress management techniques such as meditation, deep breathing, and yoga can help reduce inflammation in the gut and promote a healthy microbiome. Chronic stress has been shown to negatively impact the microbiome and disrupt gut-brain communication, so managing stress is crucial for overall gut health.

Lastly, the use of probiotics and prebiotics can also be beneficial in improving the connection between the nervous system and microbiome. Probiotics are live bacteria that promote the growth of beneficial gut bacteria, while prebiotics are non-digestible fibers that provide nourishment for beneficial gut bacteria.

Overall, improving the connection between the CNS, ENS, and vagus nerve with the microbiome is crucial for optimal physical and mental health. By focusing on a healthy diet, physical activity, stress management, and probiotic or prebiotic supplementation, we can promote a healthy microbiome and improve communication between the gut and brain.

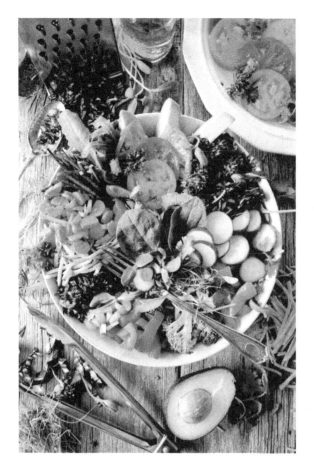

SUCCESS STORY

According to Linda (2022), Roxanne, a busy mom of four and a dedicated beauty therapist, found herself struggling to balance her family life and work, eventually leading to her neglect in taking care of her own health and well-being. As she ran around taking care of her children and tending to her clients, she found herself eating on the go and grabbing whatever was convenient rather than focusing on a healthy diet (Linda, 2022c).

Roxanne's lack of self-care soon started to manifest physically, particularly in her digestive and gut health, leading to painful abdominal cramps and bloating that lasted for weeks. Feeling increasingly uncomfortable and at a loss for a solution, Roxanne confided in a close friend who recommended Linda from Just for Tummies, a renowned digestive health expert. Linda suggested that Roxanne should start with a five-day charcoal cleanse. The activated charcoal in the cleanse works as a powerful detoxifier, absorbing the toxins and gas in the intestines, reducing bloating, and easing abdominal pain.

Within just a day of using the capsules, Roxanne had already noticed an improvement in her condition. This experience served as a wake-up call, and she realized the importance of self-care and the connection it had to her gut health. As her physical pain subsided, she became more committed to practicing self-love and attempting to incorporate activities that brought her joy and rejuvenation.

Some activities Roxanne started engaging in included indulging in a massage or a facial to help her relax, attending a yoga class for physical fitness and mental clarity, practicing meditation as a daily ritual to calm her mind, and spending time in nature by taking hikes in the woods. She also enjoyed a relaxing bubble bath on days when she needed an instant pick-me-up and made it a priority to spend some alone time to recharge her energy.

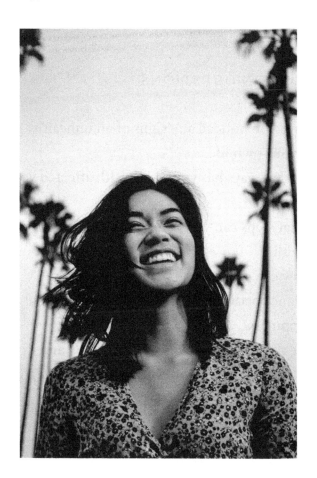

Roxanne's gut health success story is a testament to the importance of taking care of ourselves, even in the busy whirlwind of life. With the help of Linda's expertise and her newfound commitment to self-care, Roxanne could improve not only her gut health but also her overall well-being, ultimately finding a better balance between her work, family, and personal happiness.

REFLECTION QUESTIONS

- Have you noticed any signs of an unhealthy gut in your own life?
- In what ways has your gut health affected you physically?
- What steps can you take to improve your gut health?
- How can self-care help you find a better balance between work, family, and personal happiness?
- Are there any activities that bring joy and rejuvenation into your life? If so, how often do you practice them?

5

WHAT ARE YOUR RIGHTS AND HOW TO BE YOUR OWN BEST ADVOCATE

B eing your own advocate for your health is a great way to stay healthy and take charge of your well-being. You know yourself better than anyone—which makes you the best expert when it comes to understanding what feels right or wrong. As an advocate, you're in control. You decide how you take care of yourself and which treatments are right for you.

You can be your own best advocate by staying informed about your health and speaking up when something doesn't feel right. Doing research on the latest treatments, news, and developments in the healthcare field can help improve your knowledge of the medical world.

This way, if you ever have to talk with a doctor, technician, or pharmacist about a possible diagnosis or treatment plan, you'll have a better understanding of the situation. This will help you build trust with your medical team by showing them that you're engaged in the conversation and knowledgeable about what's going on.

It's true that you know your own body better than anybody else, and it's important to recognize when something doesn't feel right. You can pay attention to your daily habits and activities to help you identify changes that may be signs of a larger issue. For example, if you are usually very active and then suddenly you find yourself not wanting to leave the house or bed, this could be a sign of depression.

Many people may shy away from bringing up their health concerns with their doctor for fear of being judged or receiving bad news, but being honest with your doctor is essential for getting the necessary care and treatment needed. It's also key to keep an open mindset and listen to what your body has to tell you without judgment or criticism. Don't be afraid to ask questions, either. Being curious and asking specific questions will only help you ensure that treatment plans are tailored specifically for you.

There's no single approach to healthcare; everybody's needs are different depending on their lifestyle choices and overall health status. So it's important not only to take your own advice but also heed the advice given by healthcare professionals who understand these nuances better than anyone else. Acknowledging what feels right (or wrong) isn't always easy, but it certainly pays off in terms of long-term health benefits!

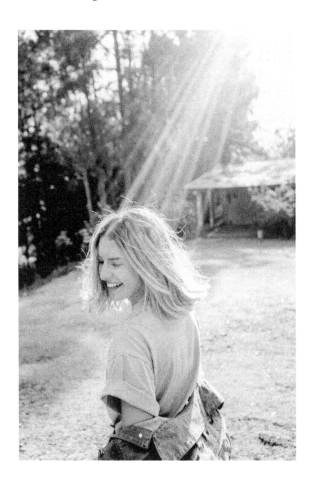

Taking charge of one's own health is empowering—and something that everyone should strive toward. When combined with regular check-ups from a doctor or healthcare provider who knows your full medical history, being an effective advocate for yourself helps create peace of mind knowing that any issue related to your health can be handled quickly and efficiently so that it doesn't become worse down the line!

YOUR RIGHTS AS A PATIENT

As a patient, it is important to know your rights in order to advocate for yourself when it comes to seeking medical care. Your rights as a patient include the right to access your medical records and information, the right to make decisions regarding your own healthcare (known as informed consent), the right to privacy and confidentiality of your medical records, and the right to receive quality care from your medical team.

Initially, knowing your rights might be overwhelming because you have much more to learn, and our rights are constantly changing or increasing as new laws or regulations are enacted. However, there are some basic rights that all patients have:

- the right to be treated with respect and dignity
- the right to receive accurate and complete information about their diagnosis, treatment options, and prognosis
- the right to access medical records
- the right to participate in decisions about their medical care
- the right to know the risks and benefits of any proposed treatments

By taking these steps and ensuring that you have access to this information, you can be an advocate for yourself and your health. Here is a breakdown of what you're entitled to and what you can ask for:

- **Access to your medical records:** You may request access to your medical records at any time as a patient. These records may include lab results, X-ray images, notes from doctor visits, treatment plans, and more. You can ask for copies of these documents or view them at the doctor's office. It is important that you understand what is in these records so that you can better advocate for yourself if necessary.
- **Informed consent:** Informed consent means that you are given all the information about a proposed procedure or treatment before

agreeing (or refusing) it. This includes any potential risks associated with receiving said treatment or procedure. Your provider must explain these risks in language that you understand before proceeding with any type of care plan. If there are any questions or concerns you have about what is being proposed, then it is important that they are addressed prior to undergoing anything recommended by your healthcare provider.

- **Privacy and confidentiality:** You may expect confidential treatment of all your health concerns and conversations with healthcare providers, including doctors, nurses, and other personnel at hospitals or clinics. The Health Insurance Portability and Accountability Act (HIPAA) ensures that certain information about a person's health status cannot be shared without their permission; this law applies whether paper-based or electronic systems are used for keeping track of health information.

- **Quality care:** Patients also have the right to receive quality care from their healthcare team —this includes clear communication from providers regarding diagnosis, preventative care measures, prescribed medications or treatments, follow-up appointments, etc.

Quality care should be provided regardless of one's race, ethnicity, or sex. If someone feels like they haven't been treated fairly based on these characteristics, then they should speak up about it!

- **Advocate for your rights:** There are many ways one can fight for their rights as a patient in a friendly manner—for example, reaching out directly with questions or voicing concerns via phone call or email with healthcare professionals who are providing care, writing letters or emails outlining specific grievances, and using social media platforms such as Twitter or Facebook groups related directly to healthcare advocacy.

Additionally, it's important to be mindful of the power dynamics in a doctor-patient relationship. Doctors are providers, and you are the patient, so it is your right to have questions answered, be heard, and be respected. If you feel overwhelmed, don't worry; making sure you are aware of your rights is a process that takes time and practice. Here are some organizations that may help empower you to become an effective healthcare advocate:

- **National Women's Health Resource Center:** This organization offers resources for women to be informed about their health and empowered to take a more active role in their healthcare.
- **American Association of Retired Persons (AARP):** AARP provides resources on healthcare advocacy, including tools to help you make informed decisions about your health.
- **Patient Advocate Foundation:** The Patient Advocate Foundation is a non-profit organization that provides medical help for patients. They provide resources on how to navigate the healthcare system, as well as legal advice and assistance with insurance matters.

Additionally, many local health departments have resources specifically designed to support women in advocating for their health. Ultimately, advocating for yourself is essential to ensure that you are getting the best care possible. Take the time to learn about your rights and find out what resources are available in your area so that you can be an effective healthcare advocate.

WHY IT IS IMPORTANT FOR WOMEN TO ADVOCATE FOR THEMSELVES AND THEIR MEDICAL RIGHTS

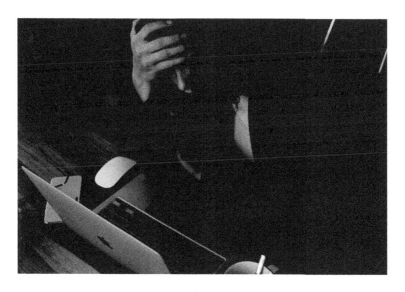

Advocating for oneself and one's medical rights is vital for everyone, but it is especially important for women. Unfortunately, women have historically faced discrimination in the healthcare system, which has led to poor healthcare outcomes and a lack of access to necessary treatments. Therefore, it is essential for women to take an active role in advocating for themselves and their medical rights.

One reason why advocating for oneself is so important is that women's health concerns are often overlooked or dismissed by healthcare providers. Women are more likely to be misdiagnosed or have their symptoms trivi-alized. This can have serious consequences, especially in cases where a timely diagnosis could be lifesaving. By advocating for themselves, women can ensure that their health concerns are taken seriously and that they receive the medical attention they need.

Another reason why advocacy is important is that women often have unique healthcare concerns that require specialized treatment. For example, reproduc-tive health issues like menstrual disorders or fertility problems may be overlooked by healthcare providers who are not well-versed in these areas. Overall this will help women ensure that they are receiving the proper care and that their healthcare providers are knowledge-able about their specific healthcare needs.

At the same time, advocating for oneself can also help women become more informed about their healthcare options, so they can make the best decisions and receive the care that is right for them. In some cases, advocating for oneself may also mean finding a new healthcare provider who is a better fit and who can provide the care and support that is needed.

Overall, advocating for oneself is an important aspect of healthcare for everyone. When women have an active role, they ensure that their voices are heard and that their medical needs are met. It is time for women to stand up for themselves and demand the care and respect that they deserve.

How Women Can Advocate for Themselves and Their Health

Your health is vital, and while doctors do genuinely care that you're well, they can only do or understand your perspective to a certain extent. As a woman, it's important to take the initiative and be vocal about your health concerns. Here are some tips for advocating for yourself and your health.

Educate Yourself

Take the time to learn more about your body, any preexisting conditions you may have, or common illnesses that are prevalent in your gender. This will help you better communicate with your doctor and understand any medical advice given to you. You've already taken a step in the right direction by reading this book and understanding the true impact that your gut can have on your well-being. Now you can not only prevent but also identify and treat any conditions you endure.

Be Proactive

Don't wait for a healthcare provider to ask you about your GI health—take the initiative to bring it up yourself during consultations. Share details about your symptoms, any dietary triggers, and your history of gut-related issues. This creates an open dialogue with your healthcare provider and emphasizes the importance of addressing your gut health concerns.

Seek Out the Right Healthcare Provider

If you feel your current healthcare provider is not taking your gut health concerns seriously, don't hesitate to search for another professional who specializes in GI health. Look for a registered dietitian, gastroenterologist, or functional medicine practitioner who has experience treating patients with your specific symptoms and conditions.

Before selecting a doctor, it's always good practice to do some research so that you are comfortable with the level of care they will offer and whether they specialize in women's health concerns, specifically before making an appointment.

Different ways you can seek a healthcare provider are

- reviews from other patients
- online databases, such as the American College of Gastroenterology's website
- word-of-mouth recommendations from family and friends

Prepare for Appointments

Before meeting with a healthcare provider, create a list of questions and concerns regarding your gut health. Bring any documentation or test results related to your gut health issues. This helps to maximize the effectiveness of your appointment and ensures you leave feeling informed and supported.

Make a List

Another way you can prepare is by making a list, putting it to the side, and adding to it every day for a week. You know your body and your symptoms better than anyone else, so take an active role when speaking to your doctor. Listen to what your body is telling you and be able to effectively explain any changes or abnormalities that you're feeling. Use the information you've learned and collected to find different ways to share your experience with your team and ask questions to ensure you receive the best care for yourself. Make sure you are an active participant in your own care.

Ask Questions

If you're concerned or confused, ask questions and voice any doubts or worries that you may have about a diagnosis or treatment plan. Remember, it's important to keep an open dialogue between you and your doctor so that you can get the best care possible. What's running through your mind right now? For example, if the doctor is prescribing a medication, it's important to ask about potential side effects or how long you should take it.

Communicate Clearly and Assertively

When discussing your gut health with healthcare professionals, be honest and clear about your symptoms and concerns. Practice active listening, ask follow-up questions, and take notes to help you remember crucial information. If you don't understand something, ask your healthcare provider to explain it in simpler terms. Remember, your healthcare provider is there to help, and it's their responsibility to ensure you understand your treatment plan.

Network With Others

Connecting with individuals who share similar gut health challenges can provide invaluable resources, support, and advice. Online forums and support groups can offer access to shared experiences and empower you to take control of your gut health.

Know Your Insurance

Navigating the complexities of your insurance coverage can be overwhelming, but understanding your benefits can help you navigate around some decision-making regarding your circumstances. Check your coverage and learn about any limits or exclusions related to your gut health treatments. Be prepared to advocate for yourself if certain treatments are not covered by contacting your insurance company and exploring alternative options.

Be Persistent

Gut health issues can be complex, and finding the right treatment approach may take time. Don't be afraid to speak up if your treatment plan isn't working or if you have concerns about your care. Remember, advocating for your gut health is a continuous process, and persistence is key.

Know when you should get another opinion. It's normal to question your doctor's diagnosis or treatment plan, and talking to other doctors can provide you with additional information. Ask your primary care doctor for their recommendation on who might be the best specialist to consult with.

Keep Track of All Medical Records

Medical records can provide valuable insight into problems or possible diagnoses, which is why it's important to keep them organized and updated on a regular basis. Be sure to ask for copies of all relevant documents, results, writeups, and labs. Even if your doctors say they will mail or fax it for you, still ask for your own copy to keep at home for your own records.

You can also keep track of your progress. Document your symptoms, treatments, and progress in a journal or digital health app. This will help you identify patterns, monitor improvements, and provide valuable information for your healthcare provider during follow-up appointments.

Request Accommodations You May Need

If there are certain types of medications or treatments that make you uncomfortable (such as narcotics), then let your doctor know so that other options can be discussed instead. Or, if you're recovering from PTSD, you can request that they walk you through each step of the visit so that you don't feel overwhelmed.

Keep Close Contact With Trusted People Who Can Help in Emergencies

Have a list of people ready who can assist in case of an emergency situation at home—friends and family members who live nearby are great resources in times like these. You should also turn to these people if you become overwhelmed or stressed. A support system is essential for health and wellness!

Don't Settle for a Treatment That Makes You Uncomfortable

If you don't feel comfortable with a certain treatment option or medication, ask your doctor what other options are available. There's no need to settle for something that makes you uneasy or may not be the best solution for your health.

Coordinate Your Care if You Have Multiple Specialists

Having multiple doctors look you over can be overwhelming and confusing, especially if they don't communicate with one another. Ask your primary care doctor to help coordinate your visits or provide a summary of the treatments or medications prescribed by other specialists. This helps ensure all doctors are on the same page and are aware of any potential risks.

File a Formal Complaint if You Feel There Is Injustice

If you feel that your doctor has acted unethically or there is injustice in the care provided, don't be afraid to file a formal complaint against them. This can help ensure that other patients are safe and taken care of in the future.

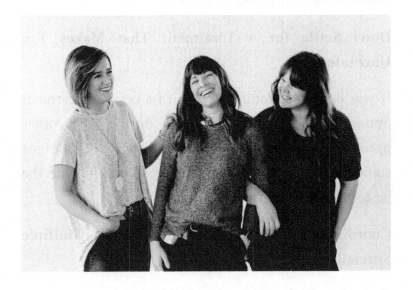

These suggestions may seem simple, but they will help you make sure that your visit with the doctor is the best it can be. Don't forget to speak up and voice your concerns if something isn't right, and don't settle for a treatment that doesn't make you feel comfortable. Remember to do your research beforehand, take notes during the appointment, and get second opinions when necessary.

WHAT TO LOOK FOR IN A DOCTOR

When women are looking for a doctor, they should consider finding someone who is knowledgeable about their health concerns, particularly digestion and gut health. These issues can have a significant impact on a woman's overall well-being, so it's essential to work with a physician who has a solid understanding of the subject matter.

In addition to knowledge and expertise, women want to feel comfortable talking with their doctor. It's essential to establish a rapport with your physician to ensure that you are comfortable discussing sensitive topics related to your health. A doctor who is approachable, compassionate, and respectful will help you feel more at ease, which will, in turn, facilitate better communication and more effective treatments.

Another crucial factor to consider is whether the doctor is willing to listen to your concerns and work with you to develop a personalized treatment plan. Women want a doctor who is willing to collaborate with them and take their input into account when making decisions about their health.

Finally, it's worth considering the doctor's availability and accessibility. A physician who is easy to reach and has flexible scheduling options can make it easier to get the care you need, particularly in urgent situations.

There are also a few technical concerns you may want to consider as well. Your insurance may or may not be accepted by your doctor, and you'll want to know ahead of time if the physician is in-network. Additionally, look at the doctor's office hours and whether they offer virtual appointments. Your health is a priority, so it is important to do your research and make sure you are working with the best doctor for your individual needs.

Overall, when looking for a doctor, you should prioritize finding someone who is knowledgeable, approachable, compassionate, willing to listen, and readily accessible. A doctor who checks these boxes can play a significant role in helping you embrace and maintain your wellness.

Surgeries for Optimal Gut Health

Gut surgeries are medical interventions that involve the manipulation of the digestive system to treat various conditions. Depending on your condition and circumstances, you may need surgery to improve your health. There are many types of gut surgeries, each with its own unique purpose and benefits. Here are some of the most common gut surgeries and what they entail (Day Kimball Medical Group, n.d.):

- **Cholecystectomy:** This surgery involves the removal of the gallbladder, a small organ that stores bile produced by the liver. Cholecystectomy is commonly used to treat gallstones, a condition characterized by the formation of small, hard particles in the gallbladder. These stones can cause inflammation, pain, and even infection if left untreated. By removing the gallbladder, the risk of further complications can be significantly reduced.
- **Colectomy:** This surgery includes removing all or part of the large intestine (also known as the colon). It is typically used to treat conditions such as colorectal cancer or diverticulitis. Colectomy may also be recommended for patients with a genetic predisposition to colon cancer or those with a high risk of developing the disease due to personal or family history.

- **Gastrectomy:** This surgery includes removing all or some of the stomach It is most commonly used to treat stomach cancer or other tumors that affect the digestive system. Gastrectomy may also be recommended for severe ulcers or other conditions that cannot be effectively treated with medication or other conservative therapies.
- **Appendectomy:** This surgery involves the appendix, a small, thin sac located at the end of the large intestine. Appendectomy is typically used to treat appendicitis, a condition in which the appendix becomes inflamed and infected. If left untreated, appendicitis can lead to serious complications, such as a ruptured appendix and a life-threatening infection.

In conclusion, gut surgeries are essential medical interventions that help to treat various conditions affecting the digestive system. While each surgery entails its own unique risks and benefits, they are all designed to help patients live healthier, more comfortable lives. If you are considering gut surgery, it is important to discuss your options with a qualified healthcare professional to determine the best course of action for your particular situation.

SUCCESS STORY

According to Guts UK, Nikki's story of overcoming IBS pain is one of success and determination. Over the course of her university days, she recognized the impact that drinking, diet, and stress had on her health (Nikki, n.d.).

As the pain became more frequent and intense due to her lifestyle choices, it gradually took over her life and forced her to take action. Nikki changed her lifestyle habits in order to manage her IBS symptoms. She cut down on caffeine, stopped drinking alcohol, and switched up her diet in order to include more fiber-rich foods.

She experimented with healthy recipes and found an appreciation for cooking. Her newfound knowledge also helped her realize the importance of exercising, proper nutrition, and looking after her mental well-being. With her new lifestyle, Nikki was able to reduce the effects of IBS symptoms in her life. This included things like managing stress better, understanding what foods help ease inflammation, learning how to eat more nutrient-rich meals and snacks, and understanding which exercises can help support your digestion.

Nikki also began sharing her IBS-friendly recipes with others in order to spread awareness about the benefits

142 | J. JOHNSON

of a healthy lifestyle for those struggling with this condition. With this newfound knowledge and dedication to self-care, Nikki could manage her IBS symptoms more effectively and lead a healthier life overall.

REFLECTION QUESTIONS

- What steps do you need to take to ensure that your doctor visit is successful?
- Are there any requests you need to make before and during the doctor visit?
- How can you keep track of all medical records?
- What should you do if you feel your doctor acted unethically?
- Who could you turn to if an emergency situation arises at home?
- Do you have an emergency plan? If not, take a moment to draft up a plan. It's important to be prepared for any situation.

6

DEVELOPING A COURSE OF ACTION FOR BETTER GUT HEALTH

A s we reviewed throughout the first set of chapters, your gut health is crucial for overall health. In this chapter, we will explore what steps you can take to improve and maintain your gut health. Having a simple course of action is important for maintaining gut health.

HABIT THEORY

The habit theory is the idea that our daily behaviors and routine actions become automatic over time. Whether we realize it or not, we create these habits through repetition and practice. Some habits can be beneficial, such as exercising regularly, while others can be unhealthy, such as overeating or smoking.

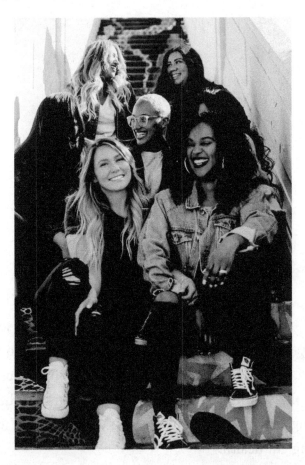

With gut health, bad habits can play a significant role. Poor dietary choices can disrupt the ecosystem in our gut. This imbalance can lead to various GI issues, such as bloating, diarrhea, and constipation.

Another example of how bad habits affect gut health is stress. Chronic stress can impact our digestive system and lead to inflammation and a weakened immune system.

If we don't acknowledge these bad habits and make a conscious effort to change them, our gut health will suffer, and we'll experience negative consequences. To improve our gut health, it's important to form healthy habits and be mindful of our actions and behaviors.

Habit Theory in Action

As women, we often struggle with habits that can negatively impact our gut health. These habits can include eating a lot of sugary and processed foods, not drinking enough water, not getting enough exercise, and not sleeping enough. However, with the habit theory in mind, we can change these bad habits and develop healthier habits that will improve our wellness and overall gut health.

The habit theory suggests that habits are formed through a cycle of cue, behavior, and reward (Orbell & Verplanken, 2020). The cue is the trigger that initiates the behavior, and the reward is the positive reinforcement that follows the behavior. By understanding this concept, we can use it to our advantage by identifying our bad habits' cues and rewards and replacing them with healthier alternatives (Orbell & Verplanken, 2020).

Let's take an example of a bad habit of eating sugary snacks when you feel stressed. The cue could be stress, and the reward could be feeling better temporarily. To change this habit, you can replace your sugary snack with a healthier alternative, such as a piece of fruit or a handful of nuts, whenever you feel stressed. This way, you still get the reward of feeling better, but with a healthier snack.

Another bad habit that can negatively impact your gut health is not drinking enough water. You should make it a habit to drink at least eight glasses of water daily. A great way to make this habit stick is to carry a reusable water bottle with you wherever you go. Keep a water bottle on hand, make sure it's always full of water, and sip throughout the day.

Finally, exercising regularly and getting enough sleep are two more critical habits that women should establish to improve gut health. Make it a habit to exercise for at least 30 minutes every day or every other day. Regular exercise can assist in digestion and reduce stress levels, which will ultimately improve gut health. Also, it is essential to get enough sleep. Try to make it a habit to turn off electronic devices an hour before bed and establish a consistent sleep schedule.

In the end, the habit theory is a powerful tool we can use to change our bad habits related to poor gut health. With tiny, incremental changes, we can make a big impact on our gut health and improve our overall wellness. By identifying the cues and rewards associated with our bad habits, swapping them with healthier alternatives, and developing new habits, we can positively influence our gut health. Remember, it takes time to develop or change your habits—be patient with yourself and stick with it.

Growth Mindset

The growth mindset is a way of thinking that focuses on personal development and the belief that ability and intelligence can be improved through hard work and dedication. This mindset emphasizes the power of effort, resilience, and determination and encourages individuals to embrace challenges and persist through obstacles. In contrast, a fixed mindset is the belief that intelligence and ability are predetermined and cannot be changed, leading individuals to avoid challenges and give up easily.

Embracing a growth mindset is crucial when it comes to improving our choices and decisions. Instead of resigning ourselves to a life of discomfort and digestive issues, we can adopt a growth mindset and empower ourselves to take action toward improving our gut health.

A growth mindset encourages us to view challenges as opportunities for growth and to keep pushing forward, even when faced with setbacks. When it comes to improving our gut health, this means not giving up if our first attempt at a new diet or lifestyle change doesn't yield the results we were hoping for. Instead, we can focus on what we learned from the experience and use that knowledge to make tweaks and adjustments until we find what works best for us.

Also, a growth mindset allows us to approach our gut health concerns with curiosity and openness. Instead of feeling shame or embarrassment about our digestive issues, we can adopt a mindset of self-compassion and understanding. This means listening to our bodies, experimenting with different approaches, and celebrating the small wins along the way.

Overall, embracing a growth mindset is essential for anyone looking to make positive changes in their life, including improving their gut health. With a growth mindset, we can approach our health concerns with a sense of empowerment, resilience, and curiosity.

DEVELOPING AN ACTION PLAN FOR BETTER GUT HEALTH

Improving gut health is an important aspect of maintaining overall wellness, as it impacts digestion, nutrient absorption, and the immune system. As a woman, understanding how to create an action plan for better gut health can be vital in supporting a healthy lifestyle. This section will help you develop an effective and sustainable plan while also explaining the importance of each step.

Evaluate Your Current Habits

The first step to creating an action plan is determining the goals you want to improve on. Begin by understanding your current state of gut health. This includes considering your diet, stress levels, exercise regime, and use of medications, such as antibiotics. Take some time to reflect on these aspects of your life and identify areas where improvements can be made. You can consult a medical professional or nutritionist or use a self-assessment health journal to track any symptoms, digestive discomfort, or irregularities. This knowledge lays the foundation from which you can build your gut health goals.

Set Realistic Goals

Now that you have a better understanding of gut health and have evaluated your current habits, it's time to set goals for improving your well-being. Make sure that these goals are specific, measurable, achievable, relevant, and time-bound (SMART) so that you can effectively track your progress and stay motivated (Mind Tools Content Team, 2022). Examples of SMART goals for gut health might include

- increasing fiber intake to 25g per day within one month
- reducing stress through mindfulness meditation for 10 minutes daily for six weeks
- drinking at least 2 liters of water each day for three months

Incorporate Dietary Changes

Make a list of healthy gut-promoting foods you can incorporate into your daily meals. This list may include probiotic-rich foods such as yogurt, kefir, sauerkraut, and kimchi, and prebiotic-rich foods like bananas, garlic, onions, and whole grains. Keep in mind your dietary restrictions and preferences, and consult a doctor or dietician if needed.

Create a Plan

With your goals set, create a detailed plan to achieve them. This plan should include actionable steps, a timeline, and resources required. For example, if your goal is to increase fiber intake, your plan could involve researching high-fiber foods, planning meals and snacks, and tracking your daily fiber consumption. When developing your plan, consider potential barriers and solutions so you can navigate challenges smoothly.

Seek Support

Improving gut health can be challenging, so seeking support from friends, family, or healthcare professionals is essential for staying on track. Share your goals with them, discuss progress, and seek advice when necessary. Maintaining open communication with your support network can keep you motivated and accountable, and it can also help you feel less alone in your journey to better gut health.

Monitor Your Progress

Regularly assess your progress and make adjustments to your plan as needed. Journaling or using a tracking app can be helpful tools for monitoring your success and keeping you focused on your goals. Reflect on your accomplishments and setbacks and remember that it's okay to encounter obstacles. Keep working on your plan to sustain gut health improvements in the long run. If you're not noticing improvements or experiencing new symptoms, you may need to reevaluate your approach or seek professional advice. Remember that achieving optimal gut health is a gradual process, and it's essential to be patient and persistent.

Celebrate Your Achievements

Lastly, take the time to celebrate your achievements throughout your journey to better gut health. Recognize the hard work you've put into making positive lifestyle changes and reward yourself when you reach milestones. This can be a powerful motivator and can help you maintain your commitment to your gut health action plan.

By following these steps, you can create an effective action plan to support better gut health, which can ultimately positively impact your overall well-being. Remember that this process requires time, patience, and persistence, but with dedication and support, you'll be well on your way to a healthier, happier you!

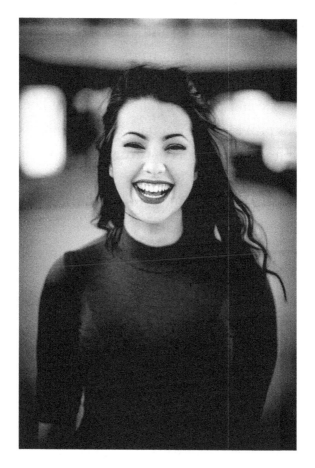

SIMPLE GOALS FOR BETTER GUT HEALTH

An action plan for better gut health is essential for women who want to achieve optimal digestive function, enhance nutrient absorption, and boost their overall well-being. Here are some attainable goals to include in an action plan to improve GI health:

- **Maintain a balanced and diverse diet:** A diet rich in various types of fruits, vegetables, whole grains, lean proteins, and healthy fats is crucial for fostering a healthy gut microbiome. These foods provide the essential nutrients and fiber that feed and support the growth of beneficial bacteria in the gut.
- **Incorporate probiotics and prebiotics:** Probiotics are live beneficial bacteria that promote gut health by populating the intestines and improving the balance of the gut microbiome. They can be found in foods like kefir, sauerkraut, yogurt, and kimchi. Prebiotics, on the other hand, are nondigestible carbohydrates that feed the probiotics, stimulating their growth and activity. Examples of prebiotic foods include artichokes, bananas, asparagus, and onions.
- **Drink plenty of water:** Adequate hydration is key to maintaining proper digestive function and maintaining the balance of good bacteria in your gut. Drinking enough water each day aids in digestion, prevents constipation, and allows the body to absorb nutrients more effectively.
- **Prioritize sleep:** Insufficient sleep has been linked to an imbalance of gut bacteria, which could lead to digestive issues. Creating a sleep-

friendly environment and establishing a consistent sleep schedule can improve both the quality and duration of sleep, ultimately benefiting gut health.

- **Exercise regularly:** Physical activity positively affects the gut microbiome by increasing the diversity of gut bacteria and promoting their overall health. Incorporating at least 150 minutes of moderate aerobic exercise or 75 minutes of vigorous aerobic exercise every week can promote better gut health.

- **Limit the intake of processed foods:** Artificial additives, high levels of sugar, and processed fats found in many processed and fast food options can create an imbalance in the gut microbiome. Limiting the consumption of these foods can help maintain healthy gut bacteria and improve overall digestion.

- **Reduce antibiotic usage:** While antibiotics may sometimes be necessary, the overuse of these medications can damage the gut microbiome, leading to various digestive issues. It's important to use antibiotics only when prescribed by a healthcare professional and to take them as directed to minimize potential harm to the gut.

By incorporating these simple goals into an action plan, women can work toward achieving better gut health, leading to improved digestion, enhanced nutrient absorption, and overall better well-being. With persistence and consistency, the benefits of these healthy habits will become evident, making it easier to maintain them as part of a regular lifestyle.

HOW TO CREATE AND STICK TO PERSONAL GOALS

Improving one's gut health is vital for overall well-being, as the benefits are numerous. As a woman, creating and sticking to personal goals for gut health improvement may be challenging but can lead to long-lasting benefits. Here, we will discuss how you can create personal goals and stick to them:

- **Identify specific gut health goals:** The first step in creating personal goals is to identify what specific aspects of your gut health you want to improve. These might include reducing bloating, improving digestion, increasing energy levels, or promoting a better gut-brain connection. By identifying specific areas for improvement, you'll be able to create more targeted and achievable personal goals.

- **Break down goals into smaller steps:** It's essential to break down your goals. Instead of going for the big picture initially, determine the smaller, more manageable steps you can take to make your goals and progress less overwhelming. For instance, if your goal is to improve digestion, begin by focusing on incorporating more fiber-rich foods into your diet, then gradually move toward additional steps like increasing your water intake, exercising regularly, or incorporating probiotics.

- **Establish a timeline:** Creating a timeline for your personal goals can help keep you on track and monitor your progress. Start with short-term goals, like making a dietary change for two weeks, then progress to more long-term objectives, such as maintaining a new habit for three months. Tracking your progress and celebrating milestones can be very motivating.

- Find accountability partners: Share your gut health goals with friends, family, or online support groups. By involving others in your journey, you'll create a sense of accountability and be more likely to stick to your personal goals.

- **Prepare for setbacks:** It's normal to experience setbacks when working toward personal goals. Instead of being hard on yourself, recognize that setbacks are part of the improvement process and use them as learning opportunities. Reflect on what caused the setback and make necessary adjustments to prevent it from recurring.
- **Make it enjoyable:** Make your gut health journey enjoyable, as you will be more likely to stick to your plans if you're enjoying the process. Experiment with new healthy recipes, find activities you love, and reward yourself for your successes.
- **Incorporate gradual changes:** Instead of making drastic lifestyle changes overnight, gradually incorporate new habits and dietary changes. This will allow your body to adjust and will be more sustainable in the long run.
- **Be patient:** Improving gut health isn't an overnight process, so it's vital to be patient with yourself. Don't be discouraged if you don't see immediate results, as it can take time for your body to adapt and for the positive effects to become apparent.
- **Remember your "why":** Remind yourself of your reasons for wanting to improve your gut

health; this could be personal, like feeling better physically or emotionally, or external, like being a healthier role model for your family. By focusing on your "why," you'll be more motivated to stick to your personal goals.

By following these steps and maintaining a positive and patient attitude, you can create and stick to personal goals that will improve your gut health and, as a result, your overall well-being.

SUCCESS STORY

According to Mind Set Health (Sexton, 2022), Sophie had endured 40 years of IBS pain and anxiety that held her back from living life on her own terms. From debilitating bloating to embarrassing gas, Sophie suffered through frequent stomach discomfort and blockages that affected her in many ways. In an effort to regain control of her health, Sophie adopted a healthier lifestyle and began practicing hypnotherapy and breathing techniques to manage her anxiety, which would often flare up and exacerbate her eating habits.

She began practicing hypnotherapy and breathing techniques in order to ease her anxiety, which had previously been exacerbating her IBS symptoms. In addition to this, she changed her diet and added more fiber-rich foods into it, as well as cutting out processed foods, alcohol, and caffeine.

After committing to these lifestyle changes, Sophie started seeing results almost immediately. Sophie was able to gradually ease the symptoms of IBS she experienced by calming the body's natural fight-or-flight response to distress. She found success in building healthy relationships with food while also learning how to effectively manage stressors in her life that could trigger unhealthy eating patterns—ultimately leading to better gut health and an improved sense of well-being.

Her IBS pain gradually decreased over time, along with the intensity of her anxiety attacks. She now has more energy than ever before and leads a much happier life than she did before. She is an inspiration to anyone who suffers from chronic gut health issues and anxiety, showing them that it is possible to live a healthy and happy life again despite these struggles.

REFLECTION QUESTIONS

- What steps can I take to improve my gut health?
- How can I identify the root cause of my symptoms?
- What dietary and lifestyle changes should I make in order to restore balance in my body?

- Am I getting enough sleep, exercise, and relaxation for optimal gut health?
- What are some small changes I can make to ensure my gut health is taken care of?
- Can I find support from friends and family members in helping me restore balance in my body?
- What other steps can I take beyond diet, lifestyle changes, and medication to keep my gut healthy?

7

THE FUTURE OF SCIENCE WILL COME FROM THE GUT

The future of science could very well come from the gut, as microbiome research continues to uncover more and more complex mysteries that have escaped our understanding before. In years to come, we can expect many exciting innovations in microbiome research. With the help of innovative technological advances, scientists can now identify each species present in the gut.

From there, they can understand how these microbes interact with one another. These advances will allow us to develop new treatments and therapies for a range of diseases and conditions that are caused by imbalances in the human microbiome. This knowledge is fundamental for developing new treatments for digestive concerns and other conditions linked to the microbiome.

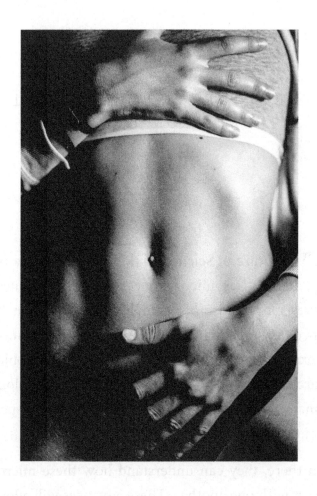

As we reviewed in the book, these bacteria can even influence how we think, feel, and behave through their connection with our nervous system (Dix, 2018). Further research in this area could lead us to discover novel therapies for mood disorders such as depression or anxiety. Not to mention, analyzing the human microbiome also helps us determine which types of foods are healthier for each individual based on their microbial composition. For example, certain probiotics may be beneficial for some people while being harmful for others due to differences in microbial ecosystems. More research in this area would allow us to pinpoint why and how this occurs, as well as how to prevent or fix it in the future.

Experts are also researching more into how gut balance can influence a person's physical and mental health. We've only begun to scratch the surface. By truly understanding the role that gut bacteria has on weight, autoimmune diseases, and even mental well-being, it's possible to unlock new treatments and preventative strategies to help people stay healthy. Innovations in this field are paving the way toward the development of personalized diets tailored specifically to an individual's unique microbial signature.

There is ongoing research into the use of fecal microbiota transplants (FMTs) to restore microbial balance in the intestines. It also counteracts dysbiosis. FMTs involve transferring bacterial material from a healthy donor's fecal sample into a patient's intestines, where it can then re-establish beneficial microbial colonies. This treatment is showing promising results so far, but further study is needed before it becomes common-place in clinical settings.

Finally, researchers are also looking at ways to exploit our understanding of the microbiota-gut-brain axis. This refers to the connection between our gut bacteria and our mental health. It's thought that treating mood disorders such as depression can be done with microbe-based interventions (Dinan, 2020). The aim here is to modulate the environment within our digestive tracts so that it supports beneficial species which produce molecules that influence our behavior positively. Although this area of research is still in its early stages, it could eventually lead us toward novel forms of psychopharmaceutical therapy.

Thanks to advances in sequencing technology, researchers will also be able to gather data on an unprecedented scale. This would allow them to make connections between changes in the microbiome and overall health outcomes that weren't previously possible. Genetic engineering techniques such as gene editing might engineer "designer" bacteria with specific capabilities. This could enable us to identify which bacteria are associated with certain health conditions or even create new probiotic strains designed for specific uses.

Overall, there's a lot of potential for exciting developments in the near future, and it's an exciting time for microbiome research. All these developments hint at an exciting future for microbiome research, one where we have a much deeper insight into how our microorganisms interact with each other and their surroundings. This would pave the way for revolutionary treatments and therapies that could revolutionize modern medicine.

As research progresses, experts hope they will identify new treatments and preventative measures that address chronic illnesses at their source: our own personal microbiomes.

MICROBIOME-BASED THERAPIES

Microbiome-based therapies aim to harness the power of the trillions of bacteria, fungi, and other microscopic organisms that live inside our bodies. Over the next few years, medical research is uncovering how these microorganisms can treat various diseases. In some cases, this involves introducing beneficial bacteria into a person's microbiome in order to restore its balance and improve health. In other cases, it may require removing harmful bacteria or fungi from the microbiome by using antibiotics or antifungals.

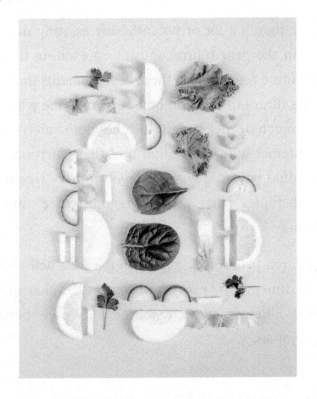

Researchers are exploring ways in which microbial communities can be manipulated to produce certain substances that can affect a person's health. For example, microbial drugs could target specific genes and disrupt processes related to disease-causing pathogens or even enhance the body's natural defenses against them. Finally, with more understanding of the links between distinct elements of the microbiome and certain conditions, researchers can develop precision therapies tailored to an individual's unique microbial community. This could lead to potentially providing new treatments for previously untreatable conditions.

For example, bacterial-based therapies are being used to treat conditions ranging from digestive disorders to brain diseases. Bacteria can deliver beneficial therapeutic compounds directly into cells or act as living drug factories within our bodies. This type of therapy is useful for targeting difficult-to-treat conditions such as cancer and Alzheimer's disease.

Another type of microbiome therapy involves using probiotics to restore balance in an unbalanced gut microbiome. Lastly, there is a new field of research known as "molecular microbial ecology." This seeks to understand how different microbes interact with each other and their environment. Doing so allows us to identify possible therapeutic strategies involving multiple bacteria strains acting together or alone. For instance, some researchers are looking at how certain combinations of bacteria might treat chronic diseases such as Crohn's disease or IBD (Dinan, 2020).

The possibilities for microbiome-based therapies seem endless. As more research is done on this fascinating topic, we will probably see even more innovative treatments emerging over the next few years that could revolutionize medicine and help us better manage a wide range of conditions.

Highly Refined Personalized Nutritional Regimes

It is expected that in the years to come, highly personalized nutritional regimes will play a major role in disease prevention based on microbiome research. Eating the right kinds of food can have a tremendous impact on your health and prevent many diseases. With advances in technology and science, we can now create even more tailored diets for individuals that consider their microbiome. Through this research, it has been discovered that certain foods can promote gut bacteria diversity, which helps to boost immunity from disease.

With highly refined and personalized nutritional regimes, you will tailor your diet to suit your unique needs. For example, if you have an intolerance or allergy to certain foods, you could adjust your diet accordingly. Additionally, by tracking what kind of food you eat and how it affects your gut microbiome diversity, you may identify any potential issues before they become serious health problems. The microbiome research could eventually provide insights into the best combination of foods and supplements tailored to each person's individual needs, offering a personalized approach that would be far more effective than one-size-fits-all dietary recommendations.

Furthermore, understanding the relationship between microbial communities and human health could help us identify which combinations of diet and lifestyle are best for an individual's overall health. For example, microbiome studies may uncover how certain dietary patterns can reduce inflammation or enhance nutrient absorption.

This information could then develop personalized nutrition plans tailored to an individual's unique health needs. Similarly, we could gain insight into how different microbes interact with one another in the human gut and how this affects our metabolism and overall health.

Ultimately, this kind of research promises tremendous potential for improving public health outcomes by allowing us to customize our nutrition plans based on our own unique biochemistry and genetics. Through increased precision in medical interventions, such as personalized diets and lifestyle guidelines, we can look forward to a future where disease prevention is more effective than ever before.

Reading Our Microbiome

The ability to read our microbiome and change it for the better is an exciting concept that is becoming increasingly realistic thanks to the amazing research in microbiome science being conducted today. In the future, microbiome research will continue to be an important area of study as scientists try to understand how manipulating the microbiome can improve human health.

Scientists are already uncovering new ways in which genes interact with the surrounding environment, including the microscopic environment inside us. Having a better understanding of how microbes interact with genes could lead to new break-throughs on how we can best treat and prevent illnesses.

This research will lead to the ability to read our micro-biome and make modifications that could potentially improve our health. By sequencing the genetic material of microbes, scientists can identify which bacteria are present in a given sample and develop therapeutics that target specific organisms.

Additionally, with advancements in gene editing tools such as Clustered Regularly Interspaced Short Palindromic Repeats (CRISPR), which can target and change specific genes in a microbe's genome, researchers can begin to develop microbial therapies that do not rely on antibiotics or other chemicals. They may also be able to modify or add beneficial genes into certain species of microorganisms that are found within our bodies.

This knowledge would enable us to directly target specific disease-causing pathogens or even introduce beneficial bacteria that can increase nutrient absorption, reduce inflammation, and regulate immune responses. Furthermore, genomic studies have identified numerous microbial metabolites that have a range of therapeutic activities, such as modulating gene expression and protecting cells from damage caused by ultraviolet radiation.

Not to mention, as technology continues to progress, it is likely that these same compounds could be developed into medicines for treating diseases like cancer and autoimmunity.

To make this technology more widely accessible for patients, researchers are developing user-friendly devices where individuals can accurately test their own microbiomes from anywhere using minimally invasive techniques. By doing so, users could track changes in their microbiomes over time and make adjustments accordingly based on professional medical advice. Utilizing this technology together with personalized treatments could allow people to better optimize their health while reducing medical costs associated with conventional treatments.

Overall, microbiome research has great potential for advancing human healthcare in terms of diagnosing diseases early on, as well as providing personalized treatments tailored toward individual microbiota profiles. With further developments in biology and bioinformatics tools, along with an increasing understanding of microbial ecology, it is likely that we will soon see increased accessibility to these technologies, allowing us to better manage our health through understanding and manipulating our microbiomes.

SUCCESS STORY

According to the IBS Coach (Waddington, 2023), Glynis had suffered from IBS for over 30 years. She had tried countless remedies and treatments to get her symptoms under control, but nothing seemed to make a lasting difference or bring her relief. That all changed when she found the IBS Coach. With the help of their specialized program, Glynis could identify the foods that were causing her symptoms and easily avoid them in her daily life. This simple practice allowed Glynis to take back control of her life and put an end to the misery of IBS taking over her life.

Now, thanks to the IBS Coach, Glynis is feeling better than ever and has been symptom-free for years. She can enjoy meals with friends and family again without

worrying about flare-ups from certain foods or ingre-
dients. She's also regained much of the energy she lost
dealing with IBS for so long and is now living a fuller,
healthier life.

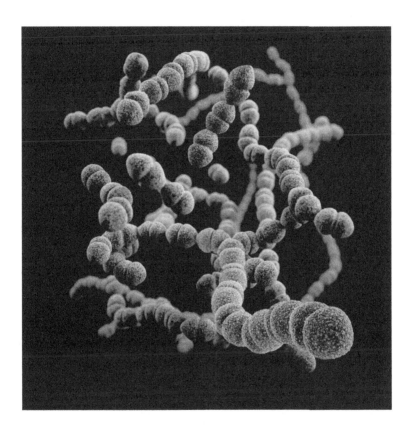

REFLECTION QUESTIONS

- How do you think the knowledge of your gut
  health can help you make positive lifestyle
  changes?

- What are some ways you can use the information about your gut health to improve your overall well-being?
- How do you think gaining knowledge of your microbiome could benefit individuals and society as a whole?
- In what ways might research in this field impact healthcare, medicine, and people being willing to speak up about their digestive concerns?
- How do you think a deeper understanding of our gut microbiomes could impact you, and society as a whole, on a day-to-day basis?

A CHANCE TO HELP OTHER WOMEN
LIKE YOU

As you start to notice the positive changes in your health and your levels of comfort, it's natural that you'll want to help other people.

Simply by sharing your honest opinion of this book – and, if you're comfortable with it, a little about your own experience – you'll show new readers where they can find the guidance they need to get their own gut health back on track.

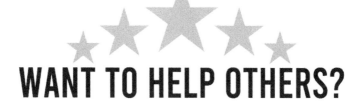

WANT TO HELP OTHERS?

Thank you so much for your support. I wish this was a subject that women were able to discuss more openly, and I want to do everything I can to help.

CONCLUSION

Congratulations! You have completed *Women and Gut Health*! So let's jump right into it. How's your poop? How are your eating habits? Has anything changed for you yet?

From the very first chapter, we reviewed the importance of gut health, and we explored the unique needs of women when it comes to their gut health. We discussed how stress and hormones can affect our digestion, and we talked about probiotics and prebiotics. We also explored some of the most common digestive issues that many women experience, along with simple lifestyle tips to help you maintain a healthy digestive system.

Can you determine, or have you already determined, which areas of your digestion need the most attention? Perhaps you can start with a few simple dietary changes or maybe some additional probiotics. Or maybe it's time to see your doctor and get a more detailed plan in place. Regardless of what you do, remember that the key to good gut health is making small, sustainable changes that you can stick with over time.

Here is a reminder of what you've learned:

- Your gut handles much more than just digestion.
- The microbiome is an incredibly complex system that plays a role in our overall health.

  ○ It consists of bacteria, fungi, and other microorganisms that work together with the digestive system to support our health.

- Women's gut health can be affected by hormones and stress, both of which can change the balance of our microbiome.
- Probiotics and prebiotics can help to restore a healthy balance in the gut, and simple lifestyle changes can help to support your digestion.

○ Common probiotics include yogurt and sauerkraut, while prebiotics can be found in foods like
bananas and onions.

- Your poop and habits can tell you a lot about
  your digestive health.

○ For example, if your stool is hard and difficult
to pass, or if you struggle with bloating and
constipation, then it might be a good idea to look
into ways of improving your gut health.

- Understanding your own body's rhythm and
  proper pooping habits can help you maintain a
  healthy digestive system for the long term.
- The gut health between men and women
  differs, and women need to be aware of their
  unique needs when it comes to their gut health.
  Some needs to be aware of are stress,
  hormones, and the balance of probiotics and
  prebiotics.

In the end, women's gut health is an important topic
that is often overlooked, and it's time that we start
taking it more seriously. With an understanding of the
microbiome and access to the right tools, you can be in
charge of your own gut health.

Behind closed doors, we were taught to be hush-hush about the yuck that comes out of our bodies. At the same time, we also needed to be more careful to avoid infections like UTIs, but this was expected of us without having all the facts and without truly realizing the power of our gut. That's why it is important to know that we have control over our digestion and overall health.

And that's why we created *Women and Gut Health*—to help other women understand and embrace their gut health.

When your gut improves, your health also improves. For instance, you may notice

- improved digestion
- better nutrient absorption
- clearer skin
- more energy
- better mental health

Before I realized the impact of my own gut health, I had been struggling with bloating and irregular bowel movements. These symptoms were worse during my period, and I was always so drained of energy.

No other women in my life were really talking about these issues—so I figured it was normal—even though my feelings resembled what was left in my toilet bowl after a heavy meal. But after learning that my health and well-being were connected to my gut health, I finally decided it was time to take control of my digestive health and make the necessary changes.

I made minor changes, such as including more fiber and probiotic-rich foods in my diet, as well as making sure I was getting enough sleep and managing stress levels. It wasn't always easy, and I definitely enjoyed the occasional cheat meal, but I saw a vast difference in my energy levels and digestive health after just a few weeks.

If you're looking for ways to improve your own gut health, here are some simple tips:

- Eat fiber-rich and fermented foods.
- Take a probiotic supplement to help boost your microbiome.
- Manage stress levels and get enough sleep.
- Avoid processed foods, added sugars, and artificial sweeteners.
- Drink plenty of water.

By taking these steps and making minor lifestyle changes, you can make a tremendous difference in your health and well-being. With the help of *Women and Gut*

Health, you can learn more about your digestive health and obtain the tools and knowledge needed to maintain a healthy balance in your gut.

Your gut is the foundation of your health, so it's important to make sure it's functioning properly. With the right diet, lifestyle changes, and understanding of your unique needs when it comes to gut health, you can take control of your digestion and improve your overall health.

We hope you feel more empowered to take control of your digestive health and make the necessary changes needed for a healthier life.

GLOSSARY

Actinobacteria: This group of bacteria is known for breaking down complex carbohydrates, like fiber, that our bodies can't digest on their own. Some types of actinobacteria, like bifidobacterium, also produce short-chain fatty acids that nourish the cells lining our gut and help keep the digestive system healthy.

Autoimmune: A condition that causes the body's immune system to mistakenly attack healthy cells and tissues in the body.

Bacteria: Bacteria are a common type of microorganism found in our gut. They play an important role in maintaining a healthy digestive system. They help the body absorb nutrients by breaking down food. They also help to protect against harmful bacteria and viruses.

Bacteroidetes: Bacteroidetes are more common in lean people. A healthy balance of these bacteria is crucial for good gut health. It helps to digest food and produce essential vitamins and nutrients.

Bifidobacteria: This group of bacteria is particularly important for infants, as they play a key role in establishing a healthy gut microbiota. They help to digest food and produce important vitamins and minerals, as well as regulate the immune system. In adults, Bifidobacteria may help to reduce inflammation and improve gut barrier function.

Bile: A fluid produced by the liver and stored in the gallbladder that helps break down fats in the small intestine.

Bolus: A mass of chewed food mixed with saliva that travels down the esophagus into the stomach.

Celiac disease: An autoimmune disorder caused by gluten that affects the small intestine. When gluten is consumed, their immune system attacks the small intestine, causing damage and inflammation. They may experience symptoms that include abdominal pain, diarrhea, and fatigue.

Central nervous system (CNS): The brain and spinal cord, which are the primary components of the nervous system that control voluntary movement, coordination, and higher-level thought. For gut health, the CNS controls digestive processes such as appetite, motility, and gut hormone secretion.

Cholecystectomy: This is a medical procedure to remove the gallbladder, which is a small organ that stores bile. It's often recommended for people with gallstones or other gallbladder problems.

Chyme: A semi-liquid mixture of food and digestive juices that moves from the stomach to the small intestine.

Clostridium difficile: A type of bacteria that can cause severe diarrhea and inflammation of the colon, often as a result of taking antibiotics.

Clustered regularly interspaced short palindromic repeats (CRISPR): This term might sound a bit intimidating, but it's actually a type of technology used to edit DNA. Scientists are researching how CRISPR can be used to study and potentially treat diseases related to the gut microbiome.

CNS: See central nervous system

Colectomy: This is a surgical procedure to remove all or part of the colon. It's often done to treat conditions like colon cancer, ulcerative colitis, or Crohn's disease.

Colon: Also known as the large intestine, it is where the body absorbs water and electrolytes from undigested food before elimination.

Commensal: Microorganisms that live in and on the human body, including in the gut. These bacteria are not harmful to humans, and in fact, they are crucial for maintaining the body's balance and health.

Crohn's disease: Crohn's disease is a chronic inflammatory disorder of the digestive tract. People may experience symptoms of abdominal pain, weight loss, diarrhea, fatigue, and other symptoms. It is thought to be caused by an overreaction of the immune system to certain bacteria living in the gut leading to inflammation and damage to the intestinal lining.

Digestion: When our bodies break down food into its component molecules, which can be absorbed and used by the body. It begins in the mouth with chewing and salivary enzymes and continues through to the stomach and intestines, where further chemical digestion takes place. The result is a nutrient-rich soup that can be absorbed through the walls of the digestive tract and delivered to the rest of the body.

Digestive enzymes: Proteins produced by certain organs (usually the pancreas) that break down food into components that can be absorbed by your gut cells for energy production or other bodily functions.

Dysbiosis: This is an imbalance between beneficial bacteria and harmful bacteria in the gut microbiome. This imbalance can cause symptoms related to GI health, such as bloating, diarrhea, constipation, gas, and abdominal pain. Dysbiosis may also be associated with other disorders or diseases, such as autism, allergies, asthma, IBD, and obesity.

Enteric nervous system (ENS): This is a network of neurons located within our digestive tract that sends signals from the brain to control muscle movements for digestion and secrete hormones that help control digestive processes like absorption and secretion of nutrients. It helps keep our intestines healthy by controlling how quickly foods move through them so we can absorb more nutrients from what we eat.

Enzymes: Proteins that help break down food into smaller molecules, which our bodies absorb. Enzymes are produced in the mouth, stomach, pancreas, and small intestine.

Escherichia coli (E. coli): Escherichia coli, or E. coli for short, is a type of bacteria that can be found in the gut. While some strains of E. coli can cause illness, most strains are harmless and actually play an important role in digestion.

Firmicutes: Firmicutes are often associated with obesity and obesity-related illnesses. They are bacteria in the gut and may contribute to metabolic diseases.

Flora: Gut flora, also known as microbiota, are the microorganisms that live in the gut. These include bacteria, fungi, and viruses. These microorganisms play a vital role in digestion, immune function, and overall health.

Fusobacteria: This group of bacteria is often associated with dental infections and other oral health issues. However, recent research suggests that they may also play a role in inflammation and other gut-related health problems (Rinninella et al., 2019).

Gastroenteritis: This is an infection in the digestive system that can be caused by viruses, bacteria, or parasites. It's often called the stomach flu and can cause symptoms like nausea, vomiting, and diarrhea.

Gastrointestinal: The gastrointestinal (GI) system comprises organs such as the stomach, small intestine, large intestine, and rectum that work together to digest our food and absorb nutrients from it. These organs are home to millions of microorganisms that are essential for proper digestion and overall health.

Gut-brain axis (GBA): The connection between the gut and the brain, where changes in one can influence the other. The GBA works to maintain a balance between physical and psychological well-being. It has been proven that disruptions to this balance can cause health issues such as depression and anxiety, to name a couple.

IBD: See inflammatory bowel disease

IBS: See irritable bowel syndrome

Immune system: The immune system is the body's defense against pathogens, such as bacteria or viruses. The gut is home to a large portion of the body's immune system, and gut health is closely tied to immune function.

Inflammation: A natural response in the immune system caused by injury, infection, or illness. Chronic inflammation in the gut can lead to health problems, including IBD.

Inflammatory bowel disease (IBD): This is an umbrella term for several chronic conditions that cause inflammation in the digestive tract. Ulcerative colitis and Crohn's disease are the most common types of IBD. Common symptoms people experience can include abdominal pain, bloody stools, or diarrhea.

Irritable bowel syndrome (IBS): A chronic condition that consists of abdominal pain, bloating, diarrhea or constipation, and other symptoms related to changes in bowel habits. IBS is often associated with an imbalance of the bacterial populations living in the gut.

Lactobacillus: This well-known group of probiotic bacteria is used to help break down lactose, the sugar found in milk, and produce lactic acid, which can help keep harmful bacteria in check. They also help to support a healthy immune system.

Leaky gut syndrome: A condition where molecules that should stay inside the digestive tract pass through the intestines into the bloodstream, causing inflammation throughout the body. Symptoms may include abdominal cramping, bloating, pain, fatigue, and skin issues like eczema or rosacea.

Microbiome: A collection of millions of microscopic organisms living in our digestive system—bacteria, fungi, and viruses—collectively known as microbiota. This microbiome affects our entire body by providing essential nutrients, helping to digest food, and fighting disease-causing microbes.

Microbiome-gut-brain axis (MGB Axis): This is an extension of the GBA, in that it explains how microbes found in the gut interact with our mental health. These microbes are essential for healthy digestion and help modulate our emotions. Studies have shown that they play a role in conditions like depression, anxiety, and stress levels.

Microbiota: This refers to the trillions of microorganisms living in our gut that are vital for maintaining gut health. These microbial communities are made up of bacteria, viruses, fungi, and archaea (single-celled organisms) that work together to help break down food particles for absorption, produce vitamins, regulate metabolism, maintain a healthy immune system, protect against bad microbes, synthesize hormones, aid digestion, boost mental health, and even influence mood.

Microorganism: Microorganisms are tiny organisms that can live in almost every environment on Earth, including in our gut. They handle many of the processes that keep us healthy such as breaking down food to extract energy and supporting our immune system.

Pathogen: A pathogen is any microorganism that can cause disease in the human body. Pathogens can include bacteria, viruses, and fungi. Some pathogens can be found in the gut, but most are harmful and can cause illness.

Prebiotics: Indigestible fibers that stimulate the growth of beneficial bacteria in the gut. Prebiotics can be found naturally in garlic, onions, leeks, artichokes, and asparagus.

Probiotics: Friendly bacteria that help to promote a healthy balance of microorganisms in the gut and aid digestion. Probiotics are found in fermented foods, such as sauerkraut, miso, and yogurt, as well as dietary supplements.

Proteobacteria: While some members of this group are beneficial, others can cause harm. For example, Helicobacter pylori is a type of Proteobacteria that can cause ulcers and other digestive problems. However, other kinds of Proteobacteria, like Escherichia coli (E. coli), are typically harmless and can even be beneficial.

Pseudomembranous colitis: an inflammation of the large intestine caused by Clostridium difficile, a type of bacteria. Treatment typically involves antibiotics such as metronidazole or vancomycin to kill the bacteria.

Sepsis: A life-threatening condition that occurs when an infection triggers a widespread immune response throughout the body. Some signs of sepsis can include high fever, rapid heart rate, low blood pressure, confusion, and shortness of breath. Early treatment with antibiotics and prompt supportive care can reduce the risk of death from sepsis.

Toxic megacolon: A syndrome where the large intestine becomes severely distended due to inflammation. It can cause severe abdominal pain, dehydration, electrolyte imbalances, and even sepsis if left untreated. Treatment typically requires aggressive resuscitation in combination with antibiotics and possibly surgery.

Vagus nerve: This long nerve runs from your brain stem all the way down through your abdomen. It acts like an information highway between your brain and your gut: it sends messages from your brain telling your gut what to do while also bringing back sensory information about what's happening inside your digestive tract to let you know if something's wrong or needs attention. This two-way communication helps regulate a variety of functions, including appetite, digestive process speed, production of stomach acids, and absorption of nutrients.

Verrucomicrobia: This group of bacteria is thought to be important for maintaining a healthy gut lining. Some types of Verrucomicrobia, like Akkermansia muciniphila, have been shown to reduce inflammation and improve insulin sensitivity, which could help prevent diabetes and other metabolic disorders.

REFERENCES

38 Hippocrates Quotes About Health, Food and Medicine. (2020, August 8). Wise Owl Quotes. https://wiseowlquotes.com/hippocrates/

Aparicio, S. (2023, January 23). *Top key gut health terminology.* Www.afpafitness.com. https://www.afpafitness.com/blog/top-key-gut-health-terminology

Bäckhed, F., Fraser, Claire M., Ringel, Y., Sanders, M., Sartor, R. Balfour, Sherman, Philip M., Versalovic, J., Young, V., & Finlay, B. Brett. (2012). Defining a healthy human gut microbiome: Current concepts, future directions, and clinical applications. *Cell Host & Microbe, 12*(5), 611–622. https://doi.org/10.1016/j.chom.2012.10.012

Barker, R. (n.d.). *The link between our gut and mental health.* Youtime.com. https://youtime.com/think/the-link-between-our-gut-and-mental-health

Bischoff, S. C. (2011). "Gut health": a new objective in medicine?. *BMC Medicine, 9*(1). https://doi.org/10.1186/1741-7015-9-24

Brabaw, K. (2016, May 18). *8 facts every woman should know about pooping.* Women's Health. https://www.womenshealthmag.com/health/a19996458/normal-pooping-habits/

Brummert, D. (2021, April 26). *Gut health: Why it matters.* Www.orlandohealth.com. https://www.orlandohealth.com/content-hub/gut-health-why-it-matters

Burba, K. (2022, August 26). *"Does your gut even need healing?": Dietitian debunks myths in trending gut health hacks.* Www.healio.com. https://www.healio.com/news/gastroenterology/20220826/does-your-gut-even-need-healing-dietitian-debunks-myths-in-trending-gut-health-hacks

Capritto, A. (2021, July 29). *How to (finally) fix your chronic stomach issues.* CNET. https://www.cnet.com/health/nutrition/chronic-stomach-issues-heres-how-to-fix-them/

Clavel, T., Horz, H., Segata, N., & Vehreschild, M. (2021). Next steps after 15 stimulating years of human gut microbiome research. *Microbial Biotechnology*, *15*(1), 164–175. https://doi.org/10.1111/1751-7915.13970

Cleveland Clinic. (2022, March 14). *Neurotransmitters: what they are, functions & types*. Cleveland Clinic. https://my.clevelandclinic.org/health/articles/22513-neurotransmitters

Cryan, J. F., O'Riordan, K. J., Cowan, C. S. M., Sandhu, K. V., Bastiaanssen, T. F. S., Boehme, M., Codagnone, M. G., Cussotto, S., Fulling, C., Golubeva, A. V., Guzzetta, K. E., Jaggar, M., Long-Smith, C. M., Lyte, J. M., Martin, J. A., Molinero-Perez, A., Moloney, G., Morelli, E., Morillas, E., & O'Connor, R. (2019). The microbiota-gut-brain axis. *Physiological Reviews*, *99*(4), 1877–2013. https://doi.org/10.1152/physrev.00018.2018

Day Kimball Medical Group. (n.d.). *General surgery*. Www.daykimball.org. https://www.daykimball.org/patient-services/general-surgery/

DerSarkissian, C. (2015, September 24). *What kind of poop do I have?* WebMD; WebMD. https://www.webmd.com/digestive-disorders/poop-chart-bristol-stool-scale

Digestive Health. (2018, July 23). *How different sexes have different digestion*. Cary Gastroenterology Associates. https://www.carygastro.com/blog/how-different-sexes-have-different-digestion

Digestive Health Services. (2022, June 8). *6 common GI problems in women*. Digestive Health Services. https://dighealth.org/posts/6-common-gi-problems-in-women/

Dinan, T. (2020, October 26). *The future of microbiome research*. News-Medical.net. https://www.news-medical.net/news/20201026/The-Future-of-Microbiome-Research.aspx

Dix, M. (2018, July 2). *What's an unhealthy gut? How gut health affects you*. Healthline; Healthline Media. https://www.healthline.com/health/gut-health

Edermaniger, L. (2019, December 31). *How to improve gut health: 16 simple hacks for your gut in 2020*. Atlas Biomed Blog | Take Control of Your Health with No-Nonsense News on Lifestyle, Gut Microbes and Genetics. https://atlasbiomed.com/blog/16-easy-hacks-to-enhance-your-gut-health-every-day-in-2020/

8 common gut health myths debunked. (2022, January 5). Atlas Biomed Blog | Take Control of Your Health with No-Nonsense News on Lifestyle, Gut Microbes and Genetics. https://atlasbiomed.com/blog/common-gut-health-myths-debunked/

EmergenC. (n.d.). *How much of your immune system is in your gut.* Www.emergenc.com. https://www.emergenc.com/newsroom/how-much-of-your-immune-system-is-in-your-gut/

Ensley, R. (2007, April). *Common GI problems in women.* American College of Gastroenterology. https://gi.org/topics/common-gi-problems-in-women/

Frost, A. (2021, December 26). *4 things about gut health even experts admit they don't know.* HuffPost. https://www.huffpost.com/entry/gut-health-experts_l_61c0b9eae4b0bb04a627fe69

GI Alliance. (2021, February 23). *Digestive disease continues to rise among Americans digestive disease continues to rise among Americans.* Gialliance.com. https://gialliance.com/gastroenterology-blog/digestive-disease-continues-to-rise-among-americans

Glossary of terms. (n.d.). The Gut Foundation. https://www.thegut.org.nz/know-the-facts/glossary-of-terms/

GMFH Editing Team. (n.d.). *Glossary.* Gut Microbiota for Health. https://www.gutmicrobiotaforhealth.com/glossary-index/

Grinspan, A. (2021, April). *C. Difficile Infection.* American College of Gastroenterology. https://gi.org/topics/c-difficile-infection/

Gupta, A. (2021, July 25). *7 digestion myths busted to deal better with your gut health.* Healthshots. https://www.healthshots.com/preventive-care/self-care/7-common-digestion-myths-that-you-must-know-about/

Health, F. (2021, July 29). *10 signs of an unhealthy gut.* Frederick Health. https://www.frederickhealth.org/news/2021/july/10-signs-of-an-unhealthy-gut/

Hi, S., & Li, H. (2021, September 28). *The gut microbiome and sex hormone-related diseases.* Frontiersin.org. https://www.frontiersin.org/articles/10.3389/fmicb.2021.711137/full

Huang, M. Y., Tang, A., & Giannini, A. (2021, June 3). *Gastroenterologists debunk 12 myths about indigestion and gut health*. Business Insider. https://www.businessinsider.com/gastroenterologists-doctors-debunk-myths-gut-health-indigestion-ibs-food-poisoning-2021-6

Krouse, L. (2020, November 24). *10 ways women can advocate for themselves at the doctor's office*. Greatist. https://greatist.com/discover/how-women-can-advocate-for-themselves-at-the-doctors

Lacy, B. E., & Spiegel, B. (2019). Introduction to the gut microbiome special issue. *American Journal of Gastroenterology*, *114*(7), 1013–1013. https://doi.org/10.14309/ajg.0000000000000303

Linda. (2022a, March 31). *"The only supplements that work!" Read Sam's story*. Just for Tummies. https://justfortummies.co.uk/the-only-supplements-that-work-read-sams-story/

Linda. (2022b, May 9). *Reduce your stress to heal your gut – Deborah's story*. Just for Tummies. https://justfortummies.co.uk/reduce-your-stress-to-heal-your-gut-deborahs-story/

Linda. (2022c, October 17). *Self-care starts in the gut – busy working mum Roxanne shares her story*. Just for Tummies. https://justfortummies.co.uk/self-care-starts-in-the-gut-busy-working-mum-roxanne-shares-her-story/

Mayo Clinic. (2020). *Gastroesophageal reflux disease (GERD)*. Mayo Clinic; Mayo Clinic. https://www.mayoclinic.org/diseases-conditions/gerd/symptoms-causes/syc-20361940

Mayo Clinic. (2021, August 10). *Celiac disease*. Mayo Clinic; Mayo Clinic. https://www.mayoclinic.org/diseases-conditions/celiac-disease/symptoms-causes/syc-20352220

McBurney, M. I., Davis, C., Fraser, C. M., Schneeman, B. O., Huttenhower, C., Verbeke, K., Walter, J., & Latulippe, M. E. (2019). Establishing what constitutes a healthy human gut microbiome: State of the science, regulatory considerations, and future directions. *The Journal of Nutrition*, *149*(11). https://doi.org/10.1093/jn/nxz154

Mind Tools Content Team. (2022). *SMART goals*. Www.mindtools.com. https://www.mindtools.com/a4wo118/smart-goals

Mulhall, K. (2021, June 25). *Success story: Rebecca 32, IBS and acne.*

Thenaturalbalance. https://www.thenaturalbalance.net/post/case-study-rebecca-ibs-and-acne

NIDDK. (2019, March 14). *National institute of diabetes and digestive and kidney diseases (Niddk).* National Institute of Diabetes and Digestive and Kidney Diseases. https://www.niddk.nih.gov/

Nikki. (n.d.). *Nikki's Story - Living with IBS.* Guts UK. https://gutschar ity.org.uk/advice-and-information/personal-stories/living-with-ibs-nikkis-story/

Oliphant, K., & Allen-Vercoe, E. (2019). Macronutrient metabolism by the human gut microbiome: major fermentation by-products and their impact on host health. *Microbiome, 7*(1). https://doi.org/10.1186/s40168-019-0704-8

Orbell, S., & Verplanken, B. (2020). *Changing behavior using habit theory* (K. Hamilton, L. D. Cameron, M. S. Hagger, N. Hankonen, & T. Lintunen, Eds.). Cambridge University Press; Cambridge University Press. https://www.cambridge.org/core/books/abs/handbook-of-behavior-change/changing-behavior-using-habit-theory/5F222BC3AF6ADD9A8307BBB726D43F5C

Pahwa, R., & Jialal, I. (2019, June 4). *Chronic inflammation.* NIH.gov; StatPearls Publishing. https://www.ncbi.nlm.nih.gov/books/NBK493173/

Paone, P., & Cani, P. D. (2020). Mucus barrier, mucins and gut micro-biota: the expected slimy partners? *Gut, 69*(12), 2232–2243. https://doi.org/10.1136/gutjnl-2020-322260

Pathak, N. (2021, October 15). *Fight for your patient rights.* WebMD. https://www.webmd.com/a-to-z-guides/health-care-21/health-care-patient-rights

Pribyl, A. (2019, May 28). *Top 10 key terms to help demystify "gut health."* Microba. https://insight.microba.com/blog/10-key-terms-to-help-demystify-gut-health/

Quin, A. (2022, February 9). *Digestive disorders affect more women than men. So why is it so hard to get a diagnosis?* Best Health. https://www.besthealthmag.ca/article/digestive-issues-gut-health-diagnosis-women-ibs-ibd-canada/

Reddy, D. (2022, May 16). *Gut health for women: Care for and feed your second Brain*. Wakemedvoices.com. https://wakemedvoices.com/2022/05/gut-health-for-women-the-care-and-feeding-of-your-second-brain/

Rinninella, E., Raoul, P., Cintoni, M., Franceschi, F., Miggiano, G., Gasbarrini, A., & Mele, M. (2019). What is the healthy gut microbiota composition? A changing ecosystem across age, environment, diet, and diseases. *Microorganisms, 7*(1), 14. https://doi.org/10.3390/microorganisms7010014

San Antonio Gastroenterology Associates. (2018, February 8). *The GI gender divide: Part I*. SA Gastro. https://www.sagastro.com/the-gi-gender-divide-part-i/

Scott, L. A. (n.d.). *Gut health and hormones*. Leigh Ann Scott MD, Las Colinas, Irving TX. https://www.leighannscottmd.com/additional-testing/gut-health-and-hormones/

Seal, R. (2021, July 11). *Unlocking the "gut microbiome" – and its massive significance to our health*. The Guardian. https://www.theguardian.com/society/2021/jul/11/unlocking-the-gut-microbiome-and-its-massive-significance-to-our-health

Sexton, C. (2022, February 16). *From IBS Pain to Empowerment: Sophie's Story*. Www.mindsethealth.com. https://www.mindsethealth.com/matter/ibs-pain

Steber, C. (2018, July 13). *11 small health symptoms women ignore, but shouldn't*. Bustle. https://www.bustle.com/p/11-small-health-symptoms-women-ignore-but-shouldnt-9696005

Stenger, J. (2021, October 5). *The rise of digestive diseases and how to take control of your gut health*. BodyBio. https://bodybio.com/blogs/blog/digestive-diseases-on-rise

Tresca, A. J. (2003, December 7). *Your digestive system and how it works*. Verywell Health; Verywellhealth. https://www.verywellhealth.com/your-digestive-system-and-how-it-works-1941716

Vann, M. R. (2015, January 5). *The 9 biggest digestive myths, debunked*. EverydayHealth.com. https://www.everydayhealth.com/digestive-health-pictures/the-biggest-digestive-myths-debunked.aspx

Vedantam, G., Clark, A., Chu, M., McQuade, R., Mallozzi, M., &

Viswanathan, V. K. (2012). Clostridium difficile infection. *Gut Microbes, 3*(2), 121–134. https://doi.org/10.4161/gmic.19399

Waddington, H. (2023). *Helen Waddington, The IBS Coach - IBS Success Stories.* Helen Waddington, the IBS Coach. https://www.theibscoach.com/success-stories/

Women and gut health. (n.d.). Dulyhealthandcare.com. https://www.dulyhealthandcare.com/health-topic/women-and-gut-health

Zoebrehob. (2022, July 5). *Common digestive issues among women.* Austin Gastroenterology. https://www.austingastro.com/2022/07/05/common-digestive-issues-among-women/

IMAGE REFERENCES

Ariadi, J. (2019, January 27). *The green apple story [Image].* Unsplash.com. https://unsplash.com/photos/QZub8Ni3x_c

Cagle, B. (2015, September 1). *Girl sitting on table with foot up [Image].* Unsplash.com. https://unsplash.com/photos/pJqfhKUpCh8

Campbell, C. (2015, October 20). *Sanctuary Cove exercise [Image].* Unsplash.com. https://unsplash.com/photos/kFCdfLbu6zA

CDC. (2020, January 23). *Computer-generated image, of a group of Gram-positive, Streptococcus pneumoniae bacteria [Image].* Unsplash.com. https://unsplash.com/photos/QEU-QgIOJKA

Cescon, G. (2018, April 20). *Blonde girl outside, looking back and smiling [Image].* Unsplash.com. https://unsplash.com/photos/00ByEXKcSkA

Cichewicz, K. (2018, February 26). *Blonde woman laying on bed [Image].* Unsplash.com. https://unsplash.com/photos/FVRTLKgQ700

Dam, M. (2017, May 14). *Closeup photography of woman smiling [Image].* Unsplash.com; Unsplash. https://unsplash.com/photos/mEZ3PoFGs_k

Jacobs, J. (2019, February 6). *Color photo of a woman's stomach [Image].* Unsplash.com. https://unsplash.com/photos/pMQgDg_8z88

Juice, D. (2018, November 27). *DOSE Juice.* Unsplash.com. https://unsplash.com/photos/sTPy-oeA3h0

Kapran, A. (2019, August 19). *Water and herbs in brown pot [Image].* Unsplash.com. https://unsplash.com/photos/p99ZKwVGBRA

Krivitskiy, A. (2019, October 7). *Black and white photo of a feminine stomach [Image].* Unsplash.com. https://unsplash.com/photos/v3jlOMgK6V8

Leunen, S. (2020, October 5). *To lay down forever sadly [Image].* Unsplash.com. https://unsplash.com/photos/G25JESFXybQ

Maridashvili, A. (2021, September 1). *Young woman looking at her reflection in the window [Image].* Unsplash.com. https://unsplash.com/photos/4VaHkL-rnZA

Mott, J. (2019, January 22). *Asian woman smiling outside [Image].* Unsplash.com. https://unsplash.com/photos/LaK153ghdig

Muniz, J. (2020, December 11). *Group of women sitting on stairs [Image].* Unsplash.com. https://unsplash.com/photos/HvZDCuRnSaY

Primeau, N. (2018, October 24). *Bowl of salad on wooden table [Image].* Unsplash.com. https://unsplash.com/photos/-ftWfohtjNw

Sims, S. (2018, January 19). *Black and white photo of a women crouched by bed [Image].* Unsplash.com. https://unsplash.com/photos/5_n3X6EfRNc

Tran, A. (2018, May 25). *Woman laying on bed with hands covering her face [Image].* Unsplash.com. https://unsplash.com/photos/i-ePv9Dxg7U

Ventur, E. (2021, May 12). *A business woman who is frustrated because she is working too much [Image].* Unsplash.com. https://unsplash.com/photos/yjHh4JpZQT8

Winger, A. (2020, February 11). *Strong women, female business owners share a laugh [Image].* Unsplash.com. https://unsplash.com/photos/Xt4g9VbMljE

Made in the USA
Las Vegas, NV
12 December 2024

13960086R00115